50TH ANNIVERSARY EDITION

HEARTBEAT

A DOCUMENTARY NOVEL MEMORIALISING
THE FIRST HUMAN HEART TRANSPLANT

Michael J. Lee

© Michael J. Lee 2020

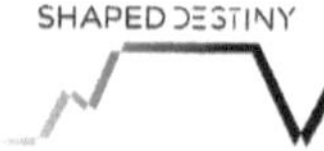

2020 Edition – First Published in 2015

ISBN 978-1-990957-74-1 (Paperback)
ISBN 978-1-990957-66-6 (eBook)

www.michaeljlee.com
www.beyondheads.com

Cover and interior crafted with love by the team at:
www.myebook.online

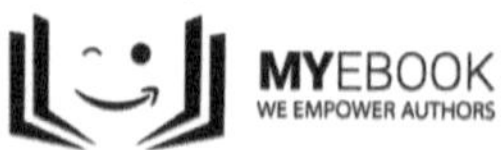

CONTENTS

*Dedicated to Professor Christiaan Barnard (1922–2001) and
Dr Marius Barnard (1927–2014),
brothers in a war against disease and injustice*

PROLOGUE

Your heartbeat times the underlying rhythm of your life. This awe-inspiring organ is the unsung hero of this real-life story and I hope you can hear it pounding inside the pages of the novel.

As a great pioneer of heart surgery, Chris Barnard, it could be said, had a heart for the human heart.

Speaking of matters of the heart, have you heard, perhaps, of Paul John Thesen? He was born on 23rd September 1965 to the Thesen family of Knysna, pioneers of shipping timber, saw-milling and forestry, and all descended from a very enterprising 19th century Norwegian settler, Charles Wilhelm Thesen. But the boy had a congenitally weak heart and, when he was fourteen, he was diagnosed at Groote Schuur Hospital as having idiopathic cardiomyopathy, a disease with no known cause. Even for one so young, there was the risk of a heart attack.

Something had to be done. So the Barnard brothers and their heart team decided to try an innovative piggy-back heart transplant, which took place on 5 January 1979. In the heterotopic procedure the team performed that day, Paul's heart was not removed but, instead, a new heart was added to his for support, giving him, in effect, a double heart. The chambers and blood vessels of the two hearts were interconnected during the operation. Thesen later had a bypass operation and, after that, a pacemaker fitted to assist his heart.

Paul John Thesen went on to enjoy a healthy and active live for another 34 years. He passed away on Christmas Day, 2013, after being found unconscious behind the wheel of his vehicle, being certified as brain-dead from a head injury on arrival at Green Acres Hospital in Port Elizabeth. He'd lived life to the full, loving the outdoors, participating gleefully in activities from sky-diving to canoeing and fishing. He also attained a brown belt in karate and took part in Paralympic games in Europe in the 1980s.

Paul had shown a great zest for life of which Louis Washkansky himself, as the first heart transplant survivor, would've been proud, and the 34 years of survival after his piggy-back transplant is a world record for heart transplants.

By a strange twist of fate, Paul was a descendant of the Thesens whose family business included wood factories where Adam Hendrikus Barnard, father to Chris and Marius Barnard, had worked as a young man, born into generations of shack-dwellers in the Knysna forest. Adam had toiled in the Thesen wood factories before moving on in 1899 from the simple woodcutter's life he'd inherited.

I guess there wouldn't have been the remarkable success story of a Paul Thesen if there hadn't been a Louis

Washkansky, and there wouldn't have been a Chris and Marius Barnard if there hadn't been an Adam Barnard determined to reinvent himself at the dawn of the twentieth century.

> How we answer the calling of our hearts echoes down the generations.

1

—————————

IMPENDING DESTINY

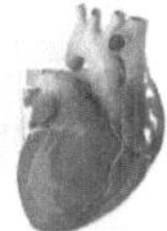

T he mid-summer sun soared in a pristine sky so bright its blue seemed to be tinged with a violet hue. Its pulsing power dominated even the rugged architecture of Table Mountain. And its light glittered and shimmered over the surface of the Atlantic which reached out into the ocean routes which had carried trade, peoples and cultures to this southern tip of Africa for centuries.

Appearing like a fortress high on the slopes of angular Devil's Peak, the state hospital of Groote Schuur towered over the suburb of Observatory and the central districts, all wrapped around the narrow strip of land squeezed between Table Bay and the city's mountainous backdrop.

It was a slow, boiling Saturday afternoon in Cape Town on the 2nd of December, 1967.

In this part of the world, weekends are always taken seriously and even the hospital's most ambitious surgeon, Professor Christiaan Barnard, was trying to relax at his lakeside home in Flamingo Crescent, Zeekoevlei, just a few kilometres from

5

the bustling, seaside town of Muizenberg which overlooks the Indian Ocean.

Destiny, though, had apparently determined that this wasn't going to be an ordinary weekend in the Cape Peninsula. When it was over, the world would no longer be quite the same place. Even as the sun blazed lazily above the city, the momentous, the seemingly miraculous, was already in the process of becoming real.

As Table Mountain stood like a monument to an elemental power, wrapped in a cloth of clouds spread by a moderate south-easter wind, a sense of impending history hung in the air. Just a few miles off this coast, within sight, Nelson Mandela, about to turn fifty, was spending his fourth year of incarceration on the bleak, inauspicious island that guarded the entrance into Cape Town's bay. In medicine, though, the field of healing, there was hope for new advances in life-extending surgery. Science had already established the knowledge and techniques required to carry out human heart transplants. A medical breakthrough was beckoning. One could almost hear the clock of history ticking.

Watching a large white pelican landing on the lake, Barnard lit another cigarette, hoping it would help him to reflect, for he was in an agitated frame of mind. With him, as he paced up and down at the bottom of his lakeside garden, were his two dogs, Ringo and Sixpence. Somewhere out on the water, which was beautifully flat, untroubled by the light wind, a seagull squalled. The breeze briefly rustled the leaves of the large Bluegums in his garden. In the lakeside shed, his boat rocked gently with the easy rhythm of the lapping water.

Barnard thought of the disagreement he'd just had with his wife Louwtjie and how she sometimes grumbled about the long hours he spent at the hospital. From his time of post-graduate study in America, it had irked him that she believed he was neglecting his family in pursuit of his career. Barnard reflected honestly on how hard it had proved to balance work commitments, personal ambitions and family obligations. He yearned for the big breakthrough he'd long dreamt about, a moment of destiny when all the vision, passion and knowledge locked up inside him would be expressed in a defining achievement. Then… everything would be different. Years of experiments, research, overseas study and ground-breaking work at Groote Schuur's cardiac unit, not to mention the sacrifices he'd made for his family, would be vindicated.

Barnard was so close and yet still so far away from his dream.

He thought about the one candidate under his supervision suitable for a possible transplant. Washkansky: the middle-aged Lithuanian Jew with a diseased heart whom everyone at the unit loved for his irrepressible humour and dogged, fighting spirit.

But the man was going downhill fast, even as his wife, Ann, left his bedside at the hospital that very afternoon and started to drive home down Main Road towards the city, the interior of her car still baking hot after standing outside for a couple of hours in the December sunshine. She was troubled by her husband's uncharacteristically low spirits. She was becoming increasingly uncertain about his chances of survival. He was starting to slide away.

"I'll see you tonight, Louis," she'd promised as she'd kissed him goodbye.

The thought occurred to her that if a heart donor couldn't be found soon, her husband would be dead before the year was out. And even if one could be found, what were the chances of success for such a radically new, untested kind of operation, one which Louis himself believed in, but which she found altogether unreal, even inconceivable?

A heart transplant.

For Barnard, too, there was plenty of anxiety on the horizon that afternoon, for the tall and handsome surgeon felt threatened by premonitions of his future as he battled against the spectre of being crippled by rheumatoid arthritis. His disease had been diagnosed back in 1956 when he was still a doctoral student in the US.

He dreaded the day his hands, which wanted to heal people, would look gnarled and useless, no longer fit for carrying out precise surgical incisions and procedures. He foresaw his career ending prematurely, his potential snuffed out by an incurable physical disability.

The surgeon was already taking pain-killers for the sharp, cramp-like contractions that sometimes shot through his hands. The uncertainties and stresses of preparing for the biggest operation of his career – the most innovative the world had yet seen - had caused recent flare-ups of arthritis in both hands and feet. From his time in America, under the mentorship of Dr. Owen "the Chief" Wangensteen, head of surgery at the University of Minnesota, the threat of arthritis – his dream-killer, his nemesis – had spurred him on to accelerate his academic progress, to aim for professional perfection, to see every opportunity for a scientific breakthrough as no less than God-given. As a proud man, he feared, above all, his ultimate decline and obsolescence.

But Barnard wasn't, by any means, a negative person. He never dwelt for long on what could go wrong. After all, he'd become used to the challenges of sickness and frailty from his days as an intern in District Six and when he'd run a general practice in Ceres. And was not Groote Schuur itself, his medical home, a battleground in the war to preserve life, health and well-being in the Cape? He'd fought his way to the top by being persistent and innovative. And hadn't his parents toiled and strained to put their sons through university, believing education to be the only way available for their family to make progress? He would refuse point-blank to let the creeping fear of arthritis threaten his future.

Besides, the surgeon believed in luck, his own luck, and in the hand of providence.

Stoking this positive mental attitude, he thought back to the successful kidney transplant he'd just carried out in September, only the second operation of its kind in his country. It gave him immense satisfaction to know that the patient, Edith Black, was recovering well.

Still, his thoughts were racing. For Washkansky was running out of time to be saved.

2

BROTHERS IN ARMS

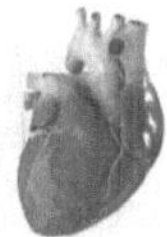

As he drew on his cigarette at the lakeside, Barnard's hazel eyes surveyed the large freshwater vlei, green with microscopic algae lit up by sunshine. As expected on a weekend, Zeekoevlei was filled with water-sport enthusiasts and anglers. Its sandy banks were dotted with country houses and boat clubs, as well as some well-positioned bird-watching hides. The doctor loved this wetlands area with its sandy fynbos and its water birds: herons, ibis, cormorants, pelicans, egrets, flamingos, kingfishers, swifts, swallows and warblers. Best of all, though, were the high-flying fish eagles. At night, he could often hear the clicking and croaking of the spotted leopard toads and arum lily frogs and the hooting of white-faced owls. It was a place alive both with nature's eco-systems and the allure of water sports: sailing, skiing, rowing and fishing.

Barnard noted with disappointment that the leaves of a wild fig tree he'd planted next to the shore had turned black from all the recent hot blasts of the summer southeaster. He made a mental note to water his fig tree more regularly or to transplant it to a shadier spot. Briefly, he thought back to the Apricot tree his parents had asked him to care for in their back garden in Beaufort West. He would've been reprimanded if that had gone to ruin. The Barnards had been taught to nurture, to exercise high levels of discipline.

He recalled moving to Zeekoevlei in the late 1950s because he'd believed, at the time, that his daughter Deirdre possessed the potential to become a world champion water-skier. He had coached her on the lake with the same intensity and drive he'd always applied to himself in his career. He thought of all the hours father and daughter had spent together out on the water, practising, drilling, always pushing the limits. He'd been a hard taskmaster to her, but hadn't he been one to himself, working his fingers to the bone to acquire his extensive knowledge and skills? How else could a person get anywhere in life? How else could he have risen above his modest provincial origins?

Barnard looked back with pride on how he'd come back from his studies in America a new and inspired man, rapidly rising to become Groote Schuur's Head of Cardiothoracic Surgery as well as Professor of Surgery at the University of Cape Town. For several years, he'd experimented, with his younger brother, Marius, transplanting animal hearts, including dozens of stray, sick dogs from the pound. There, the Barnard brothers had been supported by Hamilton Naki, a former economic migrant from the Eastern Cape with a strong natural aptitude for understanding anatomy, despite lacking a secondary school education, and who was being groomed as a laboratory assistant. Together, they'd honed their surgical skills and techniques on these outcast animals. To save humans in the long-run, they'd believed, it was necessary to let animals no one wanted carry the risks of perfecting new medical procedures and techniques.

As siblings, Chris and Marius had always been more like acquaintances than brothers. They'd never really got on particularly well, too different in nature to find enough common ground for a lasting friendship. They'd never fully bridged the five year difference between them. Chris had been their mother's blue-eyed boy, just cause on its own for the existence of some jealousy between them, which could tip over into antagonism. He even looked like his mother, Maria, with his boyish, dark-haired good-looks. But under his handsome appearance raged a brooding, even moody temperament, allied to a creative, searching intelligence.

Over the years, the Barnard brothers had sometimes ended up at loggerheads with each other, both professionally and personally. They'd grown up – and grown apart – in rough, trying times. And they themselves were tough, boys who'd often been barefoot during childhood and youth, boys who could fight, boys who'd learnt to fend for themselves, boys who could always make a little go a long way. A bit like the Karoo landscape into which they'd been born.

But in the heart team which Chris had assembled at Groote Schuur, they needed each other, even though they remained opposites, like positive and negative magnetic forces. Chris had offered his younger brother his current job when he'd needed it. To manage the periodic bickering that inevitably broke out between them, they settled on a *modus vivendi* in the cardiac section whereby Chris would operate in A Theatre and Marius would be in charge of B Theatre. And, for the most part, the system worked well.

Deep in their unconscious, though, they both knew that one of their brothers, Abraham, had been a blue baby with a sick heart. He'd constantly struggled for breath in his short two years of aborted life, an infancy characterised by physical suffering. Had they both, as a result, gravitated towards medical careers in which they could help children and adults with such life-threatening heart conditions?

And, embedded in their memories were recollections of playing Hide and Seek in their back garden, rolling tyres down the small koppie overlooking their little dam, swimming in it to cool off in the relentless Karoo summers, setting up scorpion fights in shoeboxes or just going to see matinees at the Star Cinema on a Saturday afternoon or visiting a touring circus.

Right now, Barnard really needed his brother, whom he trusted implicitly, in his team, taking care of things in B Theatre. It had to be the strongest team around if his highest career goal was ever to become reality. Everything was now in place for him to dare to carry out the world's first heart transplant; everything, that is, except a heart donor.

The surgeon thought of the risks, of all the things that could go wrong when working simultaneously with two hearts, one living and one dying. To succeed, he would need not just his knowledge and the collective expertise and experience of his thirty-strong heart team, but, somewhere inside of him, some kind of blind faith and sheer crazy guts. For he would be crossing an entirely new threshold. It would be an operation executed at a level of procedural complexity never yet accomplished.

Day by desperate day, Washkansky was fading, that brave heart of his about to pack up for good. Would time be on their side? Or would it favour the well-funded, more experienced American surgeons like Dr Norman Shumway of Stanford, Richard Lower, head of the cardiac programme at the Medical College of Virginia, or Adrian Kantrowitz of

Detroit, who were also poised to carry out human heart transplants?

Aim to be first, Barnard's devout and hard-of-hearing mother had always taught him: never second, never third. Her commitment to academic excellence from her sons had been uncompromising – sometimes even backed-up by hidings in the event of any sign of mediocrity. The brilliance of the Barnard brothers as cardiac surgeons owed much to her – as well as to the loving support of their kindly, highly principled and devoted father.

Suddenly, the surgeon felt so tired he couldn't think, or dream, any more. He'd been physically and mentally on edge for too long. He stubbed out his cigarette on the grass and, feeling spent, went inside to lie down for an afternoon nap.

What he didn't know, as he shut his eyes, is that a family tragedy had begun to unfold in the southern suburbs of the city, about twenty kilometres away, which, despite its bloody grimness, would turn the night ahead into the most incredible hours of his lifetime.

A frontier of human experience was about to open up before his eyes which had never before been breached by any one, let alone by a man secretly bearing a handicap.

3

DENNY

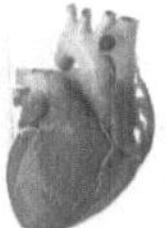

Twenty-five year-old Denise Ann Darvall, a bright-eyed, soft- faced brunette, with a silky smooth complexion and a gentle disposition, had recently bought her first car. It was a small green Ford Anglia. She loved driving around in it, demonstrating her growing independence.

A banker in Cape Town, she'd just been presented with another opportunity to show off her new toy. The Darvalls had been invited by friends to afternoon tea in Milnerton. Soon after 3pm that Saturday, they left their house in Tamboerskloof above the city bowl area. Her parents, Edward and Myrtle, were travelling in the back seat. Next to her was her younger brother Keith, aged fourteen.

On the way, Denise, known to her friends as Denny, wanted to buy a caramel cake from her favourite bakery, Wrensch Town, as her contribution to the tea. The baker was one Joseph Coppenberg, located in Salt River, renowned for his cream doughnuts and cakes.

Driving in the opposite direction from the Simonstown end, a few kilometres further ahead of the Darvalls' car, was a 36-year-old salesman and police reservist. He'd been drinking before he got behind the wheel of his shiny red Opel Cadet. He loved the sensation of speed as much as the intoxication he often fell back on to relieve the stress of a demanding, and often thankless, job.

Hearing the Monkees' brand new hit "Daydream Believer" on Radio Good Hope, his face lit up and he promptly turned up the volume:

Cheer up, Sleepy Jean, oh, what can it mean

To a daydream believer and a homecoming queen?

In Denny's Anglia, a different song was entertaining its occupants. She was singing "Lara's Theme" from the popular film *Doctor Zhivago*. Earlier that day, she'd been teaching Keith how to play the melody on the piano. The tune was still fresh in her mind. As their vehicle worked its way up Main Road in Salt River, Keith hummed along with his sister.

Then, spotting the bakery ahead, on the opposite side, Denise stopped singing and pulled over to park. Her mother got out with her, while her father and brother stayed behind in the car.

"How about half a dozen donuts as well, Darling?" pleaded Edward.

Myrtle looked at her waist and hips and shook her head.

"No, we'd better just get the cake," she replied. "Won't be a minute."

Myrtle and Denise hesitated while they waited for a break in the traffic before crossing the road. Then they disappeared inside the bakery, which was situated about one hundred metres up from where the Anglia was parked. Mother and daughter were gone for a few minutes, which seemed a long time to the occupants in the car, especially as it was starting to get roasting inside the stationary vehicle.

When the women eventually re-emerged, Denise carefully balancing the white cake box, a large truck heading towards Observatory appeared further down the road.

"There's Mom and Denny coming now," Keith said to his father, whose view of the road was obscured from his vantage point in the rear of the car.

By now, the drunk driver was travelling well above the speed limit as traffic in the direction towards the city had eased up. Distracted by the sight of the lorry, his senses and judgment dulled by liquor, he didn't notice the two women starting to cross the road. So he accelerated to pass the truck. At that moment, his vehicle smashed into the older woman with such force that her body, in turn, catapulted into her daughter, sending her flying through the air. There was a loud thud and a bang, brakes screeched, tyres screamed, someone shouted, others stood by helplessly, motorists slowed down to see what had happened. A fearful scene confronted them.

"O, Lord, there's been an accident!" Keith shouted.

"Where? Where?" Edward replied, becoming afraid.

Instead of answering, the boy got out of the car.

At that point, there was a minute in which the world seemed to stop turning, taking stock of its latest human losses. It was obvious to anyone who'd seen the collision that this was a major accident.

Myrtle's body lay motionless on the pedestrian crossing in the middle of Main Road. She'd died on impact. As Denise had fallen, her head had cracked against the back hubcap of a parked car. Then her body had rolled on the road, coming to rest in the gutter, barely alive. Blood flowed from her mouth and nose.

"Dad!" Keith Darvall yelled. "It's Mum and Denise!"

People gathered around, whispering, unsure what to do. Keith, anxiety mounting in his heart, hurried across the street, followed by his father, who was moving slowly because he was still recovering from a recent stomach operation. When Edward saw the scene in front of him, his mind went black for a few seconds and he almost toppled over. By the time he regained his senses, he found himself sitting on the pavement. Someone must have pulled him off the road so he wouldn't hurt himself. Then he remembered what was happening. But, by then, he couldn't reach his wife for all the commotion and people gathered around her body on the road. A few metres away, a cake lay splattered over the road. Both the box and cake had been trampled.

Unable to get to his wife, Mr Darvall moved towards his daughter's limp figure. It disturbed him that she was lying in the gutter. When he saw blood spattered on her head, his heart was instantly broken. He bent over to pick her up so that he could cradle her in his arms like he had often done when she was a child.

"No! Don't touch her!" a man yelled, running towards them.

The voice came from a doctor, Louis Ehrlich, who lived in the area. He'd been showering to cool off, after attending a bar mitzvah for the son of a colleague, when someone had started pounding on his door, shouting: "There's been an accident, come quick, Doctor!" He'd immediately come out of the shower and hastily thrown on a pair of pants, a shirt and his slippers. Parts of his body and his hair were still wet as he ran out into the sticky heat to respond to the call for help.

Edward stood back respectfully to let the doctor examine his daughter. Ehrlich brushed away the injured woman's moist hair and began to wipe her face with his handkerchief.

"She's still alive but deeply unconscious," the doctor announced. "But her skull has been fractured and she has severe head injuries."

Edward tried to hold his daughter again.

"No, I would leave her," the doctor advised.

The traffic police arrived and started directing vehicles away from the accident scene and instructing the crowd to get back from the road. Soon after that, Ann Washkansky, returning from her afternoon visit to her sick husband at Groote Schuur Hospital, and accompanied by her sister-in-law, Ann Taibel, drove past. A policeman waved them on.

"God, there's a woman lying in the middle of the road," Mrs Washkansky remarked.

"No, there are two of them," her passenger said. "Look!"

It was then that they recognised Ehrlich bending over the stricken woman at the side of the road. He was a doctor they both knew, prominent in the local Jewish community.

Someone from the bakery had called an ambulance at the nearest depot in Pinelands. It was 3.40 pm. Ambulance

Number 16, driven by Fred Jones Munnik and assisted by Jan Marais, was dispatched. As Munnik put on the siren, he wondered what weekend mayhem awaited him. Why did folks get so carried away just because the weekend had arrived, he thought to himself, acting silly and doing risky, dangerous things? After twenty years in the service, he'd come to the conclusion that weekends should be banned. That way, fewer people would be maimed and killed. He'd seen enough human wreckage on Fridays and Saturdays to last him a lifetime.

Four minutes later, the ambulance arrived at the scene, scattering the remaining bystanders in the road. The accident was on a smaller scale than he'd expected. He stepped down from the ambulance and approached Mrs Darvall's body. He could see she was lifeless, her body lying absolutely still. He knew a cadaver when he saw one, so still, almost like an inanimate object. Then he turned to look at Denise. She was lying on her back, her head next to the wheel of a parked car. Munnik noticed a dent in its hub-cap, indicating her head had struck it with some force, breaking her skull like a shell. He put his ear close to her face and heard her breathing heavily. She turned her head from side to side as if trying to work through the terrible concussion in her brain and to cope with all her head injuries.

"She has compound skull fracture," Dr Ehrlich told the ambulance driver. "She needs treatment as soon as possible to save her life."

"Denny! Myrtle! Speak to me! Say something, please…" Mr Darvall was calling out, wandering around in a state of shock.

Munnik and Marais wasted no time in stretchering both accident victims into the ambulance. They also decided to take the grieving man with them because he was exhibiting signs of shock and mental trauma. Keith began to look for the car keys in order to lock up the Anglia.

Munnik sped away, the siren of his ambulance blaring. He knew Denise would not live for long without life support. On their way, he called the Control Room.

"Sixteen to Control, over."

"Control to Sixteen, come in, over."

"Got two European women, one deceased and one gravely injured."

"Got you, Sixteen. Where are you taking them?"

"I'm *en route* to Groote Schuur Emergency – please inform them now."

"Will do. Over and out."

Darvall could hear his daughter moaning softly as the speeding vehicle swayed and thundered along. It took the ambulance three minutes to reach Groote Schuur's Emergency section.

Munnik and Marais unloaded Denise first, wheeling her into the Accident and Emergency section. Edward followed them, still in a daze. The duty doctor was waiting for them and he climbed onto the ambulance to check the state of the second victim. He pronounced her dead on arrival. By the time he dismounted from the vehicle, Mr Darvall had come out of emergency looking for his wife. He held on to the ambulance door to stop himself from falling over.

"Are you the husband?" the doctor asked him.

"Yes."

"I'm very sorry that your wife has died."

Darvall's legs gave way and he fainted. The doctor tried to break his fall, but failed. So Munnik and Marais lay him onto a stretcher and wheeled him into the corridor outside the emergency room where his daughter was being examined.

The ambulance then took Mrs Darvall's body to the city morgue to await an autopsy.

It did not take the medical staff long to conclude that Denise was brain-dead. One of the registrars, Dr Bertie Bosman, known simply as Bossie, confirmed her injuries were too severe for survival to be possible. Bosman was a tall, strong man with dark, wavy hair, receding from the front, matched by thick arching eyebrows protecting his ever-vigilant, rather protuberant eyes. Conscientious and sincere, he was respected and liked at Groote Schuur.

Bosman went to tell Mr Darvall the news. The doctor first helped the old man to sit down.

"Mr Darvall, I regret to inform you that your daughter cannot survive," Bosman said. "Her brain was split open when her skull was fractured by the blow to her head. She's what is known in the medical profession as brain-dead. I'm so sorry."

Darvall had already been sedated but tears fell down his cheeks once again. He loved his daughter much more than his own life, almost as much as he loved his wife.

While he was trying to comprehend his losses, two of his cousins came over to visit Denny. They offered to take him home.

"What home?" he replied. "There's nobody in it. How can I go to a home with nobody in it?"

Doctors and nurses did try to resuscitate the young woman, pumping air into her through a tube inserted into her nose. Hour after hour, they continued until most of them realised it was a hopeless task. By evening, a few hours after the drunk driver had put her life into mortal jeopardy, they finally gave up.

4

LOUIS WASHKANSKY

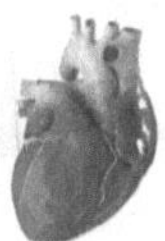

It was the chronic shortness of breath which had forced Louis Washkansky to visit his physician, Barry Kaplan, back in April 1966.

"My wife keeps thinking I'm going to die lying next to her in the bed every night because I can't breathe. It's getting bad."

"Okay, Big Fellow, let's examine you," Dr Kaplan had suggested, suspecting a deteriorating heart problem.

His patient had already experienced a heart attack the year before which had damaged the organ's left ventricle.

Kaplan had grown fond of feisty Louis and his wife. They all moved in the same social circles in the Cape's growing Jewish community. Coincidentally, they'd both originated from Lithuania.

It didn't take the physician long to arrive at a troubling diagnosis.

"As I suspected, it's not your lungs, Louis, it's your heart again."

"Darn it, what's wrong this time?"

"You have Cheyne-Stokes breathing," Kaplan explained.

"What's that?"

"You're struggling to breathe because your heart is weakening."

"What can be done?"

"I'm going to start you off on amino-phylline suppositories. That should provide relief and help you to sleep, Louis."

"I'm already taking fifteen pills a day, you know."

"I know, but you need your sleep – and your wife needs hers. This will help."

Following this prescription, there was, indeed, a brief respite for Washkansky. Soon afterwards, however, he was back for a follow-up appointment. His shortness of breath had returned and then intensified. He'd also developed an incessant cough. In addition, his legs had swollen alarmingly.

New x-rays showed an enlarged, diseased heart, bigger than Kaplan had ever seen in his life. Supposed to be the size of a fist, Washkansky's heart had become like a giant bag filling his chest. It was no wonder his ECG results had worsened. Both the left and right ventricles of his heart were deteriorating. On top of all this, the patient's liver had started to expand. As if that were not enough, his diabetes had worsened.

For Kaplan, it was, in fact, a miracle that his patient was still walking and driving around, selling his groceries and running his wholesale business as he'd always done. This was despite angina pains, fainting, breath failure and even the occasional coughing up of blood. While Kaplan marvelled at Washkansky's fighting spirit and endurance, he was compelled, reluctantly, to give him a bleak prognosis. His friend had now entered a life-and-death struggle. His spirit and his will to live were strong but his physical heart was degenerating rapidly.

"At this rate, Louis, you only have a few months to live. I'm sorry."

"Well, I'm not going to let my wife or my loyal customers down, Doc, right?"

"And you're not going to miss your Friday night soccer matches or your weekend parties, are you, Louis? I know you only too well. But I'm afraid you have no choice but to slow down and rest. I'm sending you to the cardiac clinic up on the hill for angiograms and further observation."

When Washkansky continued to go about his normal daily life, including weekend social activities, refusing point-blank to slow down, Kaplan admitted him to Groote Schuur hospital for a period of enforced rest in September, 1967.

But there was nothing that could be done to reverse Washkansky's physical decline. He even went into a diabetic coma during his hospitalisation. Not long after regaining consciousness, he suffered a stroke. This left him with hemiballismus in one hand. And when his legs filled up with liquid, medical staff inserted Southey's tubes to provide relief.

Still, Washkansky refused to die or to give up hope.

In November, after weeks of less-than-successful treatment, Professor Velva ("Val") Schrire, the small, grey-haired, bespectacled head of Groote Schuur's Cardiology, whom Barnard had been pestering for weeks for permission to carry out a heart transplant, summoned Dr Kaplan to his office.

Schrire was a pioneer of cardiology, highly respected at the hospital as a brilliant diagnostician who could pinpoint intuitively the most complex of heart conditions by listening to the history of the patient and to the sounds of their heart. He would then use x-ray and ECG results to confirm his diagnosis.

Schrire had established the hospital's cardiac clinic in the 1950s. At the time, it had been one of the first of its kind in the world. What this modest and quietly spoken cardiology pioneer told Kaplan astounded the physician.

"Look, Kaplan," he said matter-of-factly, "we're thinking of transplanting a heart into Washkansky."

Kaplan was speechless. He'd never heard of such an operation.

"How do you think your man will react to this idea?" Schrire enquired. "You know, there's absolutely nothing more we can do for him."

"Well, I'm not sure, but Louis is a fighter, a real character. He'll do anything to go on living. I know he'll take his chances for life."

"Good. Would you be so kind as to talk to him about this?"

Kaplan nodded and then excused himself from Schrire's office, still dumbfounded. He went straight over to Washkansky's ward. He found his friend smoking a cigarette, his swollen legs hanging over the side of the bed. It was the same old Louis, determined to disobey all the rules and stay in control of his own life at all costs.

"There's something we might be able to do for you," the physician told him.

"What's that, then?" Washkansky asked, feigning boredom, drawing on his cigarette.

"It's a helluva gamble and you may not come out of the operation alive."

"What kind of op are you talking about?"

"They're thinking of taking out your heart and implanting a donor heart into you."

"Hell," was all the sick man could say.

After a short pause, Washkansky looked up at Kaplan, no longer concealing his real emotions.

"I'll take it. If it's my only chance, give it to me, I'll take it," he announced, a pleading look appearing in his eyes, along with a subtle smile.

"Don't you want to think about it first? What about discussing this with Ann?"

"No, there's nothing to discuss, nothing to think about. I can't go on living like this, the way I am. It's not a life."

"Louis, I must warn you, such an operation has never been done before, anywhere," Kaplan insisted. "It could all go horribly wrong."

"Things are horribly wrong already," Washkansky responded.

Kaplan knew how stubborn his patient was, a lovable rogue always pushing the boundaries, a playful spirit you could never box in.

"I'll take the chance as soon as it comes," the intrepid grocer stated.

As a child immigrant from Lithuania, Washkansky had learnt early in life how to adapt to changing conditions and how to make the most of opportunities. As a young man, he'd taken up amateur boxing, learning how to take punches, to keep fighting even when hurt or bruised. Years of weightlifting had further toughened him up. He'd served with South African forces during World War II in campaigns in North Africa and Italy. After the war, his wholesale grocery business had steadily grown in Cape Town as he built up an extensive network of suppliers and customers, working at a tireless pace.

Kaplan looked at his friend with admiration and sorrow. Here was a man with a zest for life, someone who'd lived richly and fully but who was now face-to-face with his own mortality. He was at war with himself - his will and spirit against his body, his mind against his failing heart.

***

I am your heart, throne of your blood, seat of your life. I give blood to you. For the life is in the blood.

The blood I give is life-enriching plasma for your whole body. Each second, my muscles squeeze together in unison to pump fresh blood through your arteries, veins and capillaries.

Listen, hear your heartbeat. Thirty million beats a year, two thousand million beats a lifetime, these are the powerful contractions for your fountain of blood, a living stream soaking your body in a cleansing, liquid goodness. The blood-flow I pump, with its red blood cells manufactured in the bone marrow factories, reaches every cell to keep you ticking with the pulse of life. I squeeze and contract a hundred thousand times a day.

The life is in the blood. It holds proteins, minerals and sugars for feeding, strengthening and repairing your cells, nutrients digested from food and turned into fuel for your body. My blood plasma moves heat, too, from inside the body out to skin and limbs. And it carries the white blood cells to fight disease, engulfing and smothering germs, bacteria and viruses trying to infect the body. It has platelets to form clots to control bleeding.

I heal your body, I feed your body, I cleanse your body. My blood is your stream of life coursing on its daily sixty-thousand-mile journey through blood vessels. That's equivalent to going around earth two and a half times. What I'm all about is giving. Inside me, there's a God-given oscillator producing an electric rhythm of impulses behind each one of your golden heartbeats.

I'm the greatest machine, greater than motor or rocket engines, greater than the most marvellous engineering masterpieces.

If I live, you live; if I die, you die.

Darvall was still at the hospital, dazed but slowly starting to collect his thoughts. His sedation had just begun to wear off. He was beginning to accept that he would have to find a way to begin life over again. Yet, he'd never felt so bereft.

He sat on a wooden chair in a hospital office opposite the room where his daughter lay helpless on an operating table.

Dr Coert Venter, responsible for Washkansky during the night shift, and Bossie Bosman, entered the small office.

Venter had trained in cardiac surgery in Pretoria and was a fiercely ambitious surgeon keen to clock up as much surgical experience as possible as he moved up the medical ladder.

"May we speak with you, Mr Darvall?" Venter asked.

Darvall looked up, waiting to hear if there was anything that could be done to save his daughter.

"Mr Darvall, we can't ever bring your daughter back to consciousness," Bosman explained in a gentle tone. "Her heart is beating but her brain has been completely destroyed."

"That's pretty hard luck," was all the grieving man could say.

Then Venter stepped forward.

"Yes, but there's something that could bring some meaning to your daughter's state," he said.

"If there's no cure for her, what could that be?" Darvall enquired.

"There's a man in our care called Louis Washkansky," Bosman said. "He has an incurable heart disease. In this hospital there's a surgeon, Dr Chris Barnard, who's ready with his heart team to carry out a transplant, the first of its kind."

Bosman and Venter could see Darvall didn't yet comprehend what was being asked of him. So they decided to press on, coming straight to the point.

"We've run the tests and we believe your daughter's heart could save this man's life. We're asking you for… permission to donate Denise's healthy heart to Mr Washkansky. In addition, there's a coloured boy in urgent need of a kidney transplant. "

This request was so unusual, so beyond the pale, that it was followed by complete silence. Bosman and Venter sat down for a few minutes to give Darvall space to think about the challenge they'd presented to him.

For some mysterious reason, a light had gone on around him. He no longer seemed to be so alone. He realised, after all, that his life was not over. He thought only about his daughter. What would she have said to the doctors if her brain had still been whole?

Immediately, a flashback appeared before his consciousness. His family were celebrating his birthday at their home in Tamboerskloof. Denny had baked a cake for him. When he bent over it, he noticed she'd carved a heart into the icing, along with the words "Daddy We Love You".

A cake. A heart. A heart of love.

Then another memory flashed before his eyes. With her very first salary from the bank, she'd bought her father a new bathrobe. That was Denise. That was his girl. Always giving. And now he was being asked to give her heart away to a stranger.

These doctors wanted his daughter's heart. Darvall already knew what had to be done. He'd taken just four minutes to make his decision.

"If you can't save my daughter," he responded, "then try to save this man and boy instead."

He knew that if he said "no", he'd be hearing her voice inside his head for the rest of his life, saying "Daddy, Daddy, why didn't you help that sick man, that poor boy?"

5

DONOR HEART

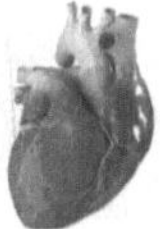

When Barnard awoke after a short nap late that afternoon, he lay for a while on his bed. He heard a speedboat roar across Zeekoevlei lake. Then he began thinking about Washkansky's dire state. He started visualising the transplant he'd been contemplating for so long. Step by step, he went through the operation, from the opening of the patient's chest. But when he came to the part in the surgical manoeuvres where he would remove the donor's heart, he saw in his mind's eye a new, less risky, way to take it out. Out of the blue, the insight came to him that he wouldn't need to cut the donor's inter-atrial septum, a step which he'd always followed in the techniques the Barnard brothers had employed in the animal laboratory and which were part of established practice reported from labs overseas, too. But the current accepted procedure carried the risk of damaging the atrio-ventricular node of the heart. Lying on his bed in the humid air, the surgeon saw no drawbacks which could result from eliminating this step. Although his idea had never been tried out before, he was convinced he'd conceived, right there and then, a genuine improvement to surgical practice for heart transplants.

Delighted by this simpler method for completing the removal of the heart, he got up from his bed and went into the kitchen to make himself some tea. Soon, the trying realities of his current situation became, once again, uppermost in his consciousness, taking the gloss off his brief moment of exultation. An impatience rose to the surface of his mind. Would Washkansky die before a donor could be found? It had been a nerve-straining wait for a donor's heart.

Impatient, Barnard decided to phone the hospital, asking to be put through to ward C-2 where Washkansky was being treated. The doctor on duty, Dr Venter, was down at casualty so Barnard spoke instead to Sister Papendieck, the most senior nursing sister in the ward, one of his favourite nurses.

"Mr Washkanksy is complaining of nausea," she told him. "And the infection in his leg is getting worse."

"How's his temperature?" Barnard asked, a trace of worry etched on his forehead.

"Stable, Professor," she replied. "And his wife was here this evening again."

"Good. He needs company. Did she smuggle in any good Jewish cooking?" Barnard quipped.

"I'd be the last to know if she did," Sister Papendieck joked, laughing.

Barnard hung up and proceeded to make himself a light supper. Louwtjie was still cross with him for all the time he kept spending away from home, including this Saturday morning, so he ate alone. After the meal, he felt weary so he returned to his bed. It was still warm.

Then, just after 8pm, the phone rang. It was Dr Venter on the line. Drowsy, Barnard half expected to hear that Washkanksy had become critical.

"Prof, looks like we've got you a donor," Venter announced.

The rate of Barnard's heartbeat increased. This unexpected news awakened his whole being: body, mind and spirit.

"Who is it?" he asked.

"A young woman. She was run over by a car this afternoon. She has severe brain damage."

"Is the girl Coloured?" Barnard asked.

The surgeon knew Professor Schrire was convinced that the international community would accuse them of experimenting with black or Coloured people if the first heart donor was not a white person.

"No, why? What's the problem?" Venter asked, nonplussed.

"Don't worry about it, I'll explain when I see you," Barnard exclaimed. "More importantly, I need to know what the neurosurgeons are saying about this donor."

"Dr Rose-Innes is examining her as we speak, Prof," Venter said.

Barnard and Peter Rose-Innes, a neurosurgeon, got on well. Both men had grown up as barefoot country boys in the Karoo, with Rose-Innes hailing from Prince Albert Hamlet near the entrance to the imposing Swartberg Pass which led to the town of Oudtshoorn.

Rose-Innes's assessment of whether or not Denise Darvall was brain-dead would be decisive.

When Barnard replaced the phone receiver, he thought the moment he'd long anticipated had probably arrived. Was this going to be the real thing, at last? But he felt far from triumphant. In fact, he became quite agitated, entering into a debate with himself. The longer he waited for the call from Rose-Innes, the more doubts seeped into his mind, so much so that he half hoped the donor would prove unsuitable after all, giving him a reprieve. He was not sure if he could make the final leap. Would his courage, or his knowledge, or even his hands, fail him in the coming moment of truth?

His mental turmoil grew to the point that he could wait no longer. So he decided to call the hospital again. Sister Papendieck answered once more.

"What's happening, Sister?"

His voice was trembling so he tried to reassert his authority by sounding matter-of-fact and even bossy.

"I'm not sure…there's no one around at the moment, Prof."

"Good grief, then, you'd better find Dr Venter," Barnard snapped. "Get him to call me."

"Ja, Professor, leave it to me."

Barnard wanted to go outside for fresh air but was afraid he'd be out of reach of the phone. He hovered over the machine, lighting another cigarette as he tried to keep himself calm. After about ten minutes, the phone rang. The ring tone seemed immeasurably louder than normal and it startled him.

"Ja?"

"There's a donor for you in C-2 ward," Venter announced.

His firm, confident tone of voice made Barnard sense things were really falling into place.

Barnard enquired about her blood group. It was O Rh-Negative.

Then he asked about consent.

"No, I haven't got consent."

This was not what the surgeon wanted to hear. He felt the blood rise up in his body, flushing his face.

"You can't just admit a patient into our ward without consent!"

On the other side of the telephone, Venter did not react to the chastisement.

"Chris, I'll find out immediately if we can get consent. This is a good donor."

These soothing words reassured Barnard.

The surgeon, gladdened, hung up, telling Venter he would come directly to Groote Schuur.

A variety of thoughts and emotions rushed into Barnard's head. The news he'd received had ended the debate he was having with himself. There was no point in further deliberations because the reality itself had already arrived. He would have to do the operation the way he was now — with what he knew, with his existing skills and techniques, with the knowledge he'd gained to this point. Destiny had come. He was like a boxer entering the ring just before the bell for round one of a world championship fight. If he won the fight, he'd be world champion, but if he lost…. He thought he might even be vilified in the international medical community. Either he was ready for this step of faith or he wasn't. He no longer had the luxury of time for reflection.

He rushed into the bedroom to put on fresh clothes. He grabbed his car keys from his bedside table. As he went out, he called out to his wife, who was still keeping to herself in his son's bedroom.

"Louwtjie – tonight could be the big night for the transplant!" he shouted gleefully.

Listening to himself say that out loud, a spurt of pride shot through him, but there was no answer from behind closed doors. Perhaps his wife was asleep?

Barnard ran through the kitchen and out to his car. It was a mere nine miles to the hospital on the hill overlooking Table Bay. Would it be nine miles to glory and success or would the night end in more tragedy? In surgery, one simple malfunction could translate, within seconds, into human loss. Those were the margins all surgeons knew so well.

Darkness had fallen at the end of a long, hot summer's day. He sped towards the hospital, sometimes driving through red lights in his haste. As he drove, in an almost dream-like state of mind, there were still so many imponderables to consider. One of the main obstacles would be getting written consent for the donor's heart. Why hadn't that been done before the donor had been admitted to his ward? And wasn't it a peculiar idea anyway, perhaps even repugnant, to put a girl's heart into a middle-aged man's body?

Although never as religious as his God-fearing parents, Barnard was nevertheless a man of prayer and faith. Alone in his car, he tried to pray, as he always did before his major operations, but this time he found words hard to come by.

He wanted to pray for the operation but it was really two operations in one, one in A Theatre and one in B Theatre. Two teams of men and women working as one in a life-and-death set of procedures.

Make each link in our chain as strong as the chain, Lord.

Please keep my hands free from pain and error.

As he drove into his parking bay at Groote Schuur, near the old main building of the hospital premises, he believed that he was coming home, that this was where he belonged, that his heart team was like his family. After all, wasn't his younger brother, Marius, an integral part of the team? Medicine was his life, healing was his calling. Always had been. This was the time and the opportunity given to him and his team. Joy and belief surged into him anew as he got out of the car and headed for the hospital's main entrance.

Lord, let me not make any mistakes. Be with my team, let us work as one heart and one mind. Walk with me now so I won't be alone.

6

CALLING IN THE HEART TEAM

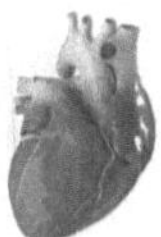

B arnard raced into the Casualty Department, looking for Venter. Inside, was the usual human carnage on a Saturday night. In a nearby ward someone screamed in pain.

The surgeon approached a nursing sister, urgency sketched on his face.

"Do you know where the heart donor is?" the surgeon asked her.

"She had a broken leg, pelvis and skull, Professor, but she's already upstairs waiting for you."

Barnard jogged up to the first floor to C-2 ward. The body of Denise Darvall lay in room 283, attended by Venter and Bossie Bosman. When he saw the victim, the heart surgeon was not happy with the fact that her legs still looked so distorted, the left leg twisted from a broken knee. The right leg was also bent, due to a broken femur and tibia.

"Can't something be done for this girl?" he asked.

Bosman and Venter looked up, confusion appearing on their faces.

"We need an orthopaedic surgeon to put her broken leg in a splint," Barnard requested.

His colleagues were taken aback.

"We must keep caring for her until the neurosurgeon says there's nothing left to do," he explained.

"Dr Rose-Innis already said as much," Bosman contended.

"Not to me, he didn't," Barnard retorted. "Please call him in for a final examination."

The surgeon then asked about consent.

"Yes, got that," Bosman confirmed, muttering to himself as he left the ward.

Barnard scrubbed himself and then slipped on a pair of surgical gloves. He and Venter worked on inserting a catheter into the saphenous vein of Darvall's right leg, running it from the groin up to the level of the abdomen. It would enable them to take blood samples, give transfusions and intravenous drugs as well as to measure pressure. She already had a tube passing through her nose into her lungs and connected to the ventilator. In addition, there were a few other tubes, including a drip for Isoprenaline to stimulate her heartbeat. In her right arm, a blood drip brought new blood into her to make up for the losses from internal bleeding which had already swollen her waist. Wires ran from electrodes on her arms and chest to an electrocardiograph machine which beeped to the echo of her heartbeat, a lonely yellow dot crossing the orange screen of the monitor.

While examining her, Barnard saw some brain tissue seeping from her left ear, a clear sign her brain had been so severely injured that there was no way back to life for her, this pretty young woman from Tamboerskloof. What had happened to Denise Darvall, the person, when she'd lost the wholeness of her brain after her head slammed against the hub-cap of the car that broke her skull? Her heart was beating but her brain was injured beyond the possibility of repair. The truth was that Denise Darvall herself would never wake up again even if her body could be kept alive for another fifty years.

What was a person without her mind? Without consciousness, the body was a human shell only.

When Barnard listened to her heart with his stethoscope, he heard a strong beat. This encouraged him. The organ was beating on blindly, pumping its own mechanical oscillator like a biological clock, still expecting to carry out its allotted lifetime of three billion heartbeats.

While he was pleased with the patient's heartbeat, Barnard had also heard the phlegmy sound of fluid building up in her lungs. He reckoned that the nasal tube would not be strong enough to drain her lungs, given the volume accumulating there.

"We need Ozzie here rightaway," he said. "Her lungs need to be sucked."

"He's apparently on his way, Prof."

"You say she's O-Negative?"

"Correct."

"We need to test the patient's acid base balance," Barnard observed. "She'll need some sodium bicarbonate and potassium. I'll also need white cell typing and cross-matching with Washkansky."

Everyone in the unit knew the surgeon was a stickler for detail with zero tolerance for any omission in procedure, any defect in absolute surgical cleanliness during operations, or for any lapse of concentration. In his presence, his theatre staff were constantly on a state of high alert. But they also knew he was as hard on himself as he was on the rest of the team. In short, Barnard was an exacting medical professional for whom only the very best was good enough.

"Critical to the success of this operation," the surgeon continued, "is a compatibility of tissues between heart donor and recipient. Otherwise, the danger of Washkansky's body rejecting his new heart would dramatically increase."

Tissue matching at the unit was carried out by Dr M.C. Botha's team of technicians at the blood transfusion service. They were due to complete the matching process in under two hours.

"We'd better get that kicked off straightaway," Barnard instructed.

"MC has already sent his girls to the lab, Prof."

"Good. Let's get some of her blood to them immediately."

He enquired about the patient's blood pressure.

"It's climbed to over seventy now," Venter explained. "We gave her an infusion."

"Get it up to ninety at least," Barnard replied. "Let's try to keep it around ninety. That'll be the safest."

His preliminary examination of the donor completed, Barnard sifted through the information and reports in her folder. He noted she was free of disease. That ticked another box. And her chest x-ray showed no signs of pulmonary tuberculosis. Another tick. Confidence was starting to pulse through his veins. He began to see the way clearing ahead of him to perform the transplantation. But they were not ready yet, not by a long chalk.

The neurosurgeons had scribbled notes on a chart tracing the rapid decline and death of her brain. Barnard was well aware of the complex legal definition of death still pertaining in the country where he'd learnt so much about organ transplantation – the United States. There was not yet the criterion of brain death to fall back on there, it had to be the whole body that was dead, heart included.

Barnard also knew legislation was more favourable to them in South Africa, since death could be determined by an official agreement between at least two practising professional doctors. Nevertheless, the operation he was about to perform would have international repercussions, so the heart team wanted to abide by prevailing medical principles.

In his own mind, Barnard regarded the brain as the body's control centre, without which it was not possible to live a proper human life. When Denise Darvall's head had crashed against a hub-cap, her ability to be herself had been taken from her. Her personhood had been stolen, even though her biological life had survived in its most basic form.

While Barnard was flipping through the patient's folder, Bossie returned with some bad news. He'd brought a cardiographic print-out from the clinic. It showed a dip in the patient's Q-R-S complex.

"Her electrocardiogram shows some irregular beats," Bosman explained, handing the results to Barnard.

The Q,R and S waves showed how regularly a heart was beating and could indicate damage to, or weakening of, the organ if they became irregular or inconsistent. Each heartbeat was like the tick of a watch – behind it was a complex machine producing a set of mechanical motions. Up to five different kinds of waves could be detected in the beating of the heart, although the three main ones were called Q,R and S.

Bosman's report worried the heart surgeon.

"Professor Schrire must see this. The rhythm of her heart could've been disrupted by the brain damage, of course. But I'm not taking out a bad heart only to replace it with an injured one. The last thing I need now is some sort of heart arrhythmia!"

For Barnard, the electrocardiogram was an important window into the heart of the patient. He could not bring himself to give Washkansky, after all the pain and sickness he'd been through in the last few years, a poorly performing heart, one with any sign of abnormality.

"Get the Prof to check this out, please," Barnard ordered, his confidence that the operation would go ahead temporarily ebbing once again.

"I'll call the whole thing off if her heart is weakening," he declared.

Dr Rose-Innis had still not arrived at the unit, so Barnard decided to find Professor Schrire himself, asking Bossie to locate the head neurosurgeon instead.

Barnard wanted clearance on the brain death and the health of the donor heart before proceeding. So far, he had neither in his hands.

At this point, he wondered if he should call in the rest of his heart team from all over the Cape Peninsula, especially since it was a Saturday night. They could be at restaurants, parties, movies, shows, having braais with friends or already sleeping. It would take a couple of hours to bring them all in.

But what did all that social activity matter in the end? It was all trivial. For the clock of history was ticking, louder and louder, as if it had its own heartbeat, its own inexorable rhythm.

Barnard decided there was no more time to waste.

"Call the full heart team in," he instructed.

That evening, his brother, Marius Barnard, and his wife Inez, were celebrating their 16th wedding anniversary with friends at their new home in Newlands, a short walk away from the suburb's rugby and cricket grounds. Marius and his guests had been wining and dining. Nonetheless, his brother summoned him to come immediately to theatre.

After he'd phoned his brother, Barnard spoke to Sister Papendieck, who was checking the urine output of the donor patient.

"Good output," she stated. "I've also checked the charts and her drips. What else do I need to do, Prof?"

"Nothing more at this point, thank you."

Barnard then left the ward in search of Schrire to discuss Darvall's all-important cardiograph. As he was leaving, his eye caught a little bunch of violets in a drinking glass next to

Denny's bed. Why hadn't he noticed them before? What was important is that someone who loved her, and cared about her, had sent them in the hope that she would be returned to life. The stranger who'd sent them probably couldn't quite imagine the world without her in it.

But Barnard knew her eyes would never see the violets given to her, because they would never open again. What remained of her life had already been given away by her father to someone else. A giving, loving woman was still giving… even while dying.

The heart specialist took one of the violets and put it in his pocket for luck.

"ARE YOU READY?"

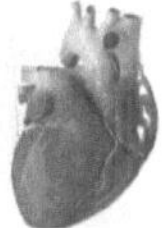

While Dr Venter and a nurse were preparing Washkansky for the operation, Barnard went to see his patient. As he walked along the corridor of C-2 ward, he was still thinking about the sacrifice of Darvall's young life before she'd even reached her prime.

Right now, he wanted to feel the conviction flow through his veins that he was doing something great on behalf of a victim who would never again speak for herself. He wanted to hear some encouragement from the mouth of his heart patient. He needed to reinforce his desire to perform an operation that would eventually save countless lives, one that would be his gift to the world. Deep down, though, he was seeking approval from God for what he was about to do. The violet in his pocket had been a small sign. Now he wanted another sign.

Near where Denise Darvall and Louis Washkansky were being treated, a doctors' office was located. There, Barnard met his staff each day to discuss patients and upcoming operations. He stopped off at the office to call Schrire, who promised to come over immediately. Then the ever-reliable Sister Papendieck came in to inform him that Dr Rose-Innis had begun his examination of Miss Darvall.

Things had begun to accelerate. Soon after that, Dr Ozinsky reported that he'd passed a larger intratracheal tube through the donor's mouth as requested. Ozzie, as he was affectionately known, was on his way to see Washkanksy, so Barnard decided to go back to the donor's room in the ward.

Ozinsky, of Polish descent, was a highly respected cardiac anaesthetist who was always impeccably polite and calm, a pillar of competence and grace. Yet underneath the gentle persona and quiet confidence was a steely determination to achieve success for each of his patients.

He was to be supported in B Theatre by a second anaesthetist, Dr Cecil Moss, a former Springbok rugby player and coach.

Barnard knew that without a healthy heart from Miss Darvall, and without confirmation from Rose-Innis that she was a brain-dead person, there wasn't going to be any transplant that night. When he re-entered her room, Dr Rose-Innis was bent over her body peering through an ophthalmoscope into the pupils of her eyes.

"What do you see?" Barnard asked.

"Her pupils are fixed and dilated, exactly as they were at five thirty this afternoon," the neurosurgeon answered. "Her brain registers no activity or response."

To support this view, he showed Barnard an x-ray of Darvall's skull. The fractures extended right across. The whole brain had shifted from the impact of the deadly blow.

"Our tests show her brain has died," Rose-Innis concluded.

Barnard was taken aback by the definitive clarity of the neurosurgeon's pronouncement. This meant the operation to remove her heart for the transplant could go ahead.

A pregnant silence followed. Both men knew what this meant.

Firstly, it was the end for Miss Darvall. There was no hope left of restoring her to life. Secondly, she had now been handed over to the transplant team. The medical goal was no longer to save her. It was to save Washkansky - through the gift of her heart. For that to happen, the team had to keep it in as perfect a condition as possible.

The two men from the Karoo wondered if Denise would've given her consent if she'd been able to speak. It had taken her father only four minutes to decide to give his permission. He'd reasoned this act would have been in keeping with who his daughter was, the young women who had driven out of her way to buy a special cake to give to her friends that afternoon. There could be little doubt that she would've supported her father's courageous decision to donate her organs.

Barnard pondered the ethics of this decision. He knew his every act would be under scrutiny if he succeeded in performing the world's first heart transplant. His point of view was that if the donor's brain was, indeed, irreparably destroyed, she couldn't live a normal human life again, and would never wake up again as a sentient woman. Denise Darvall was in a limbo that was like a living death. She'd been robbed of her personhood, which was her humanity. No doubt she could be kept alive artificially, hooked to machines and tubes, in a vegetative coma, for several years. The surgeon believed that medical resources had to be used to save viable human lives, not to prolong a dehumanised existence in this state of arrested death.

Barnard and Rose-Innis both knew Denise Darvall was in a twilight state between life and death. The life-giving partnership between brain and heart had been severed, leaving her with an existence without life.

For so many years as a surgeon, the Barnard brothers had been operating at this threshold of life and death. Sometimes, it was a haunting place to be. Sometimes, there was only was a thin margin between the two states of the body. Now, however, the donor had crossed over the point of no-return into her ghostly intermediate state. What Barnard wanted to do was take the life still lingering in her heart and kidney so that some of her dying body would be transferred to those most in need.

Professor Schrire came to examine the donor. He looked at her x-rays and cardiographs. While pondering the results, he was quiet, reflective.

"The dip in her cardiograph was caused by brain damage," he announced. "Her heart is good, Chris, it's ready for transplant. But the longer you wait, the more damage there could be to this organ."

Barnard was elated, relieved that he had the official go-ahead for the operation.

He immediately set off to see his patient. Washkansky was lying back as his bare chest was being shaved in preparation for being cut open.

"Hello, Doc, I guess this is it?" he asked, his eyes searching the face of his benefactor for assurance.

The surgeon smiled.

"Yes, Louis, this is it. Are you ready?"

"I'm kinda ready, kinda shaky."

"That's natural, don't worry," Barnard told him.

"What's my opponent like today?" Washkansky enquired, reverting to a favourite boxing analogy.

At first, Barnard didn't know what to say. No one really knew what death itself was like, not even a surgeon.

"I'm in your corner with you all the way," he said, after a few moments.

"But the odds…what are my odds now, just before tonight's fight?"

"They're moving in your favour, but…."

"But what, Doc?"

"It's not going to be easy in the ring."

"I'll take my odds, Mr Heart Surgeon. Just tell my wife it's in the bag so she doesn't need to worry about a thing."

"Alright, will do."

Washkansky and Barnard looked into each other's eyes for any signs of anxiety or pre-fight nerves. In their mutual respect and admiration, an atmosphere of trust had been built up. Neither man saw any fear.

Barnard promised to check in one more time before the operation began and then left. He went into the doctor's office to call Mrs Washkansky. He informed her they had a donor and were ready to proceed with the transplant.

"Louis told me to tell you not to worry, it's in the bag."

"Thank God. Professor, is it really in the bag for my husband?"

"We'll do our best. We have more than a fifty-fifty chance."

"Thank God," she repeated.

Barnard had fulfilled his last duty and all the hurdles had been surmounted. It was time to get scrubbed up and ready for the long and complicated operation.

Unexpectedly, at that moment, a wave of uncertainty assailed him and he found himself face to face with an old enemy – doubt.

8

COMPLETING THE CIRCLE OF LIFE

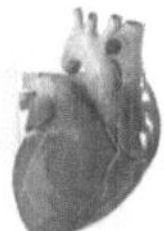

Striding down the corridor to the operating theatre just after midnight, the reality of what was happening hit Barnard hard. It felt like his knees were turning to jelly. Things were happening too fast. He wanted to turn back the clock, but it was too late.

As Denise Darvall and Louis Washkansky were being wheeled into adjacent operating theatres, the heart surgeon knew he was now locked into an unfolding history. His relentless drive towards innovation and experimentation had brought him to this point.

What lay before him in the two interlocking operating theatres? Both the donor and the patient were depending on him and his heart team to succeed: Darvall to make her death count for the world and Washkansky to reverse his own descent into death.

Barnard remembered the story in Genesis about making Eve from the rib of Adam. Now it was the organ of a woman that could bring life to a man, giving him a second chance to live and complete his circle of life.

But last-minute doubts and fears threatened to overwhelm Barnard. Wasn't it too soon to try such an audacious procedure? What if he failed, if his hands cramped up in arthritic contractions?

Was his team really ready?

He thought back to the number of dogs which had died at the animal lab after experimental heart transplants. And now he wanted to try this on humans? It was a fearful prospect.

Doubt was an old enemy in the Barnard psyche. He'd grown up in a home of modest means in a small dusty railway country town surrounded by the dry, silent, rocky beauty of the Great Karoo.

His father had been the missionary to the Coloured folk of Beaufort West at the Dutch Reformed Mission Church. In those days, in the heyday of apartheid, it was a divided town. Many times, his family had endured mockery, intolerance and prejudice. The parsonage at 77 Donkin Street had been spacious but humble, without hot running water, telephone, television or indoor bathroom.

Money had been scarce in their home. Had not three of the four surviving sons, namely, Johannes, Chris and Marius, needed study loans from the Afrikaans charity Helpmekaar to assist them to pay for their university education? Had they not sometimes worn hand-me-downs? During his medical studies, Chris had been forced to stay with his married brother Johannes in Pinelands, walking miles every day in all weather conditions to attend lectures and tutorials at the University of Cape Town.

Yet even this simple lifestyle in the Karoo town had been a step-up from the social conditions in which previous generations of Barnards had lived. Chris's father Adam had come from a long line of woodcutters dwelling in the forests of Knysna in times before there were any roads leading in, or out, of it and when wild animals and elephants still roamed freely.

These forest-dwelling Barnards had been low-income whites living in their corrugated iron and wooden homes without running water or electricity. They had felled trees, especially stinkwood and yellowwood, and then cut up the timber, selling it to monopolistic timber agents who'd regularly exploited them. They were largely uneducated people who'd lived and died simply by the words of the Holy Bible.

Through an extraordinary effort of will, Adam Hendrikus Barnard, whose own parents had never left the forest, had ventured into the world beyond it to seek a better life for himself and his descendants. He'd joined the Salvation Army in Oudtshoorn and eventually worked his way up in the church to become a minister of religion. Afflicted all his life by severe asthma, he'd then served his congregation faithfully for 37 years. He was as tough and as gentle as the succulents dotting the Karoo veld around their home.

But whatever the Barnard home may have lacked in finances, it was rich in ethics, a household strong in values and in humanity. An instinctive love for fellow humans, irrespective of origin, race or social status, flowed strongly through the Barnard bones.

For as long as he could remember, Chris Barnard had possessed a burning ambition to prove his worth to the world, spurred on by his memories of scarcity and struggle.

But now, suddenly, on this strange Saturday evening, when his moment of truth had arrived in the big city hospital, everything seemed too pressing and enormous for him. Wasn't he out of his depth? And weren't the risks he was taking just too high, given the current level of medical knowledge about heart transplants?

The presence of doubt in his mind at this crucial moment was distressing, especially since it was on a scale he'd never before encountered in his career. He decided he needed to pray – and soon. *Nood leer bid.*

He came to the dressing room door marked Medical Staff Only. There, each member of the team would shower, scrub their hands and arms, using an antiseptic solution to kill off surface germs. After that, they would apply antibiotic ointment to their nostrils. Finally, they would cover their faces and hair and put on their germ-free linen scrubs and rubber boots.

Inside, he entered the first locker room reserved for junior surgeons and registrars. Some members of the team were stripping to shower, including Marius, his brother, who would help remove the donor's heart. Everyone turned to look at Barnard, forcing him to hide his mixed emotions and put on, instead, a brave face.

"We'll prepare the donor to go on the by-pass machine in case there's any heart failure, right?" Marius asked Chris.

"Right."

"And we'll wait for you to give the go-ahead before we open her up, okay, Chris?"

"Yes," their leader replied, not in the mood for talking.

"Then you come in and excise her heart."

"Don't you want to do that?" Barnard asked.

"No."

"Why ever not?"

"Remember with the dogs, Chris, it's better if you cut the heart out yourself so you're not dealing with a heart you don't know."

"Right, right," Barnard agreed. "I should've thought of that."

He was grateful to Marius for this insight and advice, but all he really wanted to do was to be alone so he could find peace of mind. He had to find out if it was right to go ahead with the operation. He had to examine his own heart, to find a source of courage deep inside him for the medical and mental battle that lay ahead that night.

He went through the second door marked Senior Surgeons. He was alone, at last. He went up to his locker. He began to undress, until he was wearing only his tartan underpants. Then he sat down in a nearby armchair, his brain a fountain of thoughts shooting in all directions. You'd better be damned sure you know what you're doing…This is simply enormous. Human lives are at stake, not animals. Louis Washkansky. Denise Darvall. It's the very purpose of medicine that's at stake here. Do you really know what you're doing? Who are you to make such life-and-death decisions? You said there was an eighty percent chance of success. Wasn't that false? Who do you think you are? Do you think your career and reputation will even last a day longer if this all fails?

Whilst wrestling with his thoughts, Barnard thought of an analogy. When your back is against the wall, there's no choice left but to face outwards. That was the position he was in. The only direction left was forward.

Sitting in the locker room, Barnard knew he was facing in the right direction. His life had come naturally to this moment. There was no turning back. His guidance from above had come – just in time, in the very last moments before the operation began. He would stay true to himself, to what he believed – about himself, about his profession. He knew he could do this because it was right to proceed, right in all conceivable ways.

"Professor Barnard?"

Someone was calling him. It was a female voice and it sounded at that moment like an angel calling his name.

"Professor Barnard," the voice repeated. "May I come through, please?"

He looked up from his armchair to see Sister Tollie Lambrechts peering around the rear door of the dressing room. He was so lost in thought it did not even occur to him to cover up his semi-nakedness. After all, this was a hospital, the place where you saw everything, where there were very few human mysteries left.

"I have the second pump to take through into B Theatre," she said, referring to the heart-lung machine to be used on Denise Darvall.

Barnard recognised the familiar old machine immediately. It had been a farewell gift to him from Professor Wangensteen after he'd completed his studies at the University of Minnesota in 1958. He'd personally brought it back with him from Minneapolis. Seeing the machine made him smile, many warm-hearted memories brought back to mind. It was the technology which had enabled him to begin open-heart surgery. It was a special moment because he was reminded of how far he'd come in the years since his return from post-graduate study in the USA. He was no student now. He was no rookie. He had done all his homework. He had gained all the required knowledge. He and his brother had worked tirelessly in the animal lab, aided by the nimble Naki and lab leader Victor Pick, experimenting with transplantations. And he had the technology needed to pull off the medical feat. He had the best heart team in the world. Yes, he, Professor Christiaan Neethling Barnard, was ready.

Peering down at himself, he realised Sister Lambrechts must have found his appearance amusing.

"Bring it through, Sister," he said, smiling self-consciously.

Emboldened, Barnard got up and opened the door to the second dressing-room. Dr Bosman was there, towel around his waist.

He asked his colleague to find someone to accompany Sister Lambrechts.

Then, looking around, he felt power flooding into him, a renewed confidence. He was also filled with a growing motivation.

"What are we waiting for, boys?" he called out.

Then, in the shower, Barnard was finally able to pray.

Lord, please guide my hands tonight, keep them free from error. Thank you for defeating my enemy doubt. Please heal this dying man and be with each member of my team every step of the way.

After these reverent moments, the heart surgeon felt encouraged.

By now, it was after midnight.

Following an invigorating shower, the surgeon pulled on white undergarments, pants and the sleeveless surgical shirt, as well as a pair of sterile rubber boots marked with his name. He walked across the corridor and marched into the operating suite. The two adjacent theatres, B for the donor and A for Washkansky, were connected by two small rooms. There, Barnard smeared neomycin ointment in both nostrils and grabbed a cap and face mask and headed for A Theatre.

Dr Ozinsky had already brought the heart patient in for the induction of anaesthesia, close to the heart-lung bypass in case his heart gave way after the administration of the drugs.

Washkansky was sitting on the table with some pillows behind his back as if this was just another room in the ward.

"Where have you been, Doc?" he asked, a trace of petulance in his voice. "Everyone has gone fishing in this place."

"I left my rod at home," Barnard quipped. "It's weekend, remember."

The surgeon noticed how hard it was for Washkansky to even talk. His joking was all part of his typical hospital bravado, expressed in banter and jokes, to which the staff at the unit were used. In reality, though, he was a very sick man.

"I didn't want your staff slipping me a Mickey Finn before I could say goodbye properly," he whispered.

Barnard was once again touched by the humour and humanity of the man he was trying to save. Washkansky was loved in the hospital for his bravery and strong character.

This was what medicine was all about, Barnard thought to himself. Already buoyant after his shower and his inner reassurances, the surgeon felt his heart overflowing with affection and care. At 45, he knew he was in the prime of his career, a depth of knowledge matched by strength, energy and aspiration.

"Goodbye?" Barnard queried, good-naturally.

"Goodbye to a sick Washkansky…"

"And hello to a new man," the surgeon added.

"Am I really going to get a new heart?"

"Yes, a beautiful, fresh heart of hope."

"So, it's out with the old and in with the new…like they say in Auld Lang Syne."

"It's not quite New Year's Eve but we'll get there," Barnard replied, smiling behind his face-mask.

Sister Fox-Smith and Dr Ozinsky allowed Washkansky to sit up in order to help him breathe while they prepared for the induction. Green blood pressure cuffs had been fastened to both of his upper arms in addition to the silver electrodes strapped to his lower arms and to his left calf. Leads from the electrodes dangled up to the electrocardiograph monitor.

"Please lie back now, Mr Washkanksy," Sister Fox-Smith instructed.

"Can't I just sit up?" he pleaded, not quite ready to fully surrender himself into the hands of the medical team caring for him.

"No," she answered.

"You have to recline," Dr Ozinsky emphasised. "These surgeons are worse than celebrities, they don't want you to be in their limelight."

Ozinsky was renowned for his humane ways, always managing to keep his patients calm and as relaxed as possible. And yet the task ahead for him demanded a high degree of vigilance – continuously checking indicators like blood pressure, cerebral reflexes, venous pressure, respiration, acid level, pulse rate and urine output.

Sister Fox-Smith removed the supporting pillows and the patient lay back in what was an act of surrender and trust. He was giving himself into the hands of Barnard's heart team. Soon, he would lose consciousness – and any control over proceedings. He would wake up either a new man in this world or as a soul departed to the next world. This was a big moment.

Ozinsky put the oxygen mask over the patient's nose and mouth.

"Just relax and breathe in slowly," he instructed.

Washkansky nodded in acceptance, looking up at Barnard, whom he trusted with his very life. Suddenly, a look of pleading appeared on his face, a trace of tears watering his eyes.

"I told Ann it's in the bag," Barnard reassured him.

Ozinsky injected a barbiturate to anaesthetise Washkansky. His eyes closed almost immediately. The man with the fighter's heart was now as helpless as a baby. The theatre wall clock read: 12.55 a.m.

The patient was then injected with a muscle relaxant. His body was now in a deep sleep. The anaesthetist inserted a tube through his mouth and down his throat and windpipe as he planned to keep him ventilated through a manual resuscitator before switching to an automatic respiration machine.

While Washkansky was still paralysed from the dose of Scoline, tubes and leads were lodged into his body to ensure sufficient ventilation, and to pick up any secretions that could clog up his lungs. Ozinsky also placed an electrothermometer through the mouth and down the oesophagus near to the right atrium of the heart to monitor the organ's temperature throughout the transplant. But the meticulous preparations weren't yet over. Dr Francois Hitchcock came in to insert a catheter into the patient's bladder for readings on urine flow as well as blood flow through the body. The less damage there was to organs and muscles during the operation, the greater would be the chances of a full recovery.

Ozzie continued pumping the bag to provide ventilation for Washkansky and to keep him asleep, with a mixture of oxygen, nitrous oxide and halothane. Then he hooked up the tube from the bag into the Bird respirator to automate the ventilation, freeing himself from this mechanical function.

Members of the surgical team and nursing staff then took final steps to get the sleeping patient ready. They strapped him firmly to the operating table. They linked him to a diathermy machine which would enable electrosurgery, that is, using electric currents passed through the surgical tools cutting the blood vessels and tissue. It would also make it easier to cut and would help the blood to coagulate after the cutting. Barnard was known as a master surgeon: this was part of his perfectionism.

Washkansky was painted with iodine to kill off surface bacteria. He glistened in a golden brown sheen as if he were sunbathing at Camps Bay or Clifton beach. He was covered in a sterile sheet and draped with theatre towels, with only his chest and right groin exposed for surgery.

Washkansky was now so connected to medical devices that he was effectively man and machine, and no longer just a man.

Barnard wanted his team to know exactly what was happening deep inside the patient's body throughout the complex operation. All these tubes and devices opened up windows into the interior of his body, allowing the medical staff to read the story of how he was responding to each surgical procedure. The patient was now ready. But what about the donor in B Theatre?

9

HEARTBEAT OF HUMANKIND

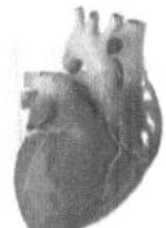

Barnard walked through the two narrow rooms connecting the theatres, the setting-up room for sterilising and checking surgical instruments and the scrub room for surgeons. Back in B Theatre, he was startled to see the donor lying with outstretched arms on the operating table where arm rests had been attached on either side. From Denise's arms, ECG leads and feed lines led up to the I.V. pole where they were hooked. For a moment, Barnard thought it looked like she was on a cross and, in a way, she was. Wasn't she giving the last portion of her life to the dying man in the adjacent theatre? Through her father's brave consent, given in the midst of intense grief, her final act of life had become a sacrifice. Sisters Amelia Rautenbach and Sannie Rossouw were painting her with iodine.

Dr Johan de Klerk, from the Karl Bremer hospital, was standing by, ready to remove the donor's kidneys for a Cape Coloured boy in his own late-night, life-saving operation. But Barnard immediately established that the heart was to be cut out first.

"De Klerk can get his kidneys afterwards," he declared.

Barnard, whose father had fought for decades against racial prejudice, relished the fact that there was no apartheid in his operation tonight, no dividing lines of race, gender or age, or any barriers between Jew and Gentile. Inside of all humans was the same heart that beat, the same red blood flowing with life. Tonight, there would be healing. Tonight, there would be justice. Tonight, his land would do a great thing for the world, for all its peoples. Tonight, all hearts were red-blooded and the heartbeat of humankind would beat as one. The grand purpose of medicine would be to heal any human in dire need. He and his team were ready to strike a big blow against heart disease.

As Marius Barnard and consultant surgeon, Terry O'Donovan, were working under the intense glare of the operating light, to get ready for the opening of the donor's chest, Barnard checked the ECG monitor. He didn't like what he saw.

Dr Coert Venter, who had hooked up drips for keeping the donor's heart in a fresh condition, told him that her condition had worsened. Her body temperature was 39, her blood pressure at 95 and her pulse rate was 100.

These were readings of a body fighting just to stay alive long enough to perform its final duty, a body starting to malfunction. Barnard was particularly worried about any damage to her heart in the next critical hour or two. Worst case scenario right now would be heart failure. Her biological clock might shut down and then the big night in Cape Town's major hospital would descend into a routine surgical failure.

With the added urgency of the donor's weakening condition, the theatre clock seemed to tick all the louder. Under its watchful eye, the clock of Darvall's heart was, indeed, slowing down. It was losing its strength, running out of ticks. Quickly, thought Barnard, we have to move very quickly now. A race against time had begun in earnest.

"Terry, get ready to open the chest and go on the pump as fast as possible," he instructed.

He knew the only way to save her heart, so that it could live inside Washkansky, was to connect her circulation to a heart-lung machine, thereby stabilising it. This support would cool down her bloodstream, putting a brake on her metabolism. Such a step would, in turn, relieve her heart's workload.

Barnard himself began to feel mental pressure mounting in him. It seemed to be pressing in on him from all sides. It was as if the clock on the wall were watching his every move, ticking ever louder to remind him that one slip of the hand, one misplaced step in the procedures, and the daring operation he'd planned throughout the 1960s could descend into tragedy.

There was a particularly delicate timing issue to get right: both hearts had to be ready at the same time. Only when he'd seen the donor's heart exposed in full flesh and blood, performing normally, and only when the recipient's heart was ready to be removed altogether, without risk to the patient, could he proceed to cut out her heart and place it into Washkansky.

In the scrub room, Barnard's chief assistant for the operation, Dr Rodney Hewitson, a Fellow of the Royal College of Surgeons, was putting on his surgical gown. He'd been summoned at that late hour from his Hermanus holiday home by police radio. A quiet, reserved and religious man, Hewitson was regarded by some as the best, most experienced surgeon on the team and indispensable for the success of the coming operation.

"Sure glad to see you, Rodney," Barnard said, relieved.

He told his right-hand man that there was no time to waste, given the donor's deteriorating condition.

Hewitson, a man of few words and impeccable professionalism, simply nodded. Calmly, he entered A Theatre to join Hitchcock. As they prepared to make their first important incision of Washkansky, the heart-lung machine, able to by-pass the patient's diseased heart and his lungs, stood ready like a silent guardian of life. Without it, no heart transplant could even take place. To succeed, the world's first heart transplant would require a combination of high-tech, the latest medical knowledge and honed surgical skills of the highest order.

Immediately, the two surgeons began opening up the patient's right groin to insert two catheters. One was to measure the venous pressure of blood returning to the right side of the heart. The other was placed in the femoral artery to hook up Washkansky's arterial system to the life-saving machine.

During surgery, cleansed blood would be fed into him from the machine but instead of entering his heart, it would hit a blocking clamp and then be forced to flow through the body in a dynamic detour. Then the blood, returning from suffusing the tissues of the body, would be siphoned back to the heart-lung machine by two other tubes inserted into the superior and inferior venae cavae. This by-pass system would keep Washkansky's body perfused with blood while the heart and lungs had been disconnected from his body's own circulatory system.

Once Washkansky was ready to be hooked up for by-pass, Barnard returned to B Theatre. Again, the news was not positive.

"I don't like the look of her," Marius Barnard stated.

Terry O'Donovan told him there had been some internal bleeding. Other indicators confirmed a downward trend. Pressure started mounting. Mental pressure, time pressure, moral pressure, even blood pressure. Pressure producing tension, in the muscles of the neck, down the spine, and in the forehead, tension squeezing down to the restless fingertips.

The respirator keeping Denise Darvall's body alive clicked and hummed. Barnard decided to stimulate the donor's heart with a dose of Isoprenaline. Marius supported switching off the respirator so Denise would stop breathing and the heart could be removed while it was still in its best shape.

"We must wait for the heart to stop though," Terry asserted.

Barnard always felt his responsibility lay first and foremost with the patient, more than with the donor.

"No, wait!" the heart surgeon decided. "Let's get Washkansky open and hooked to by-pass first. Then you can switch off the respirator. I don't want her heart to be damaged in any way if there's an unexpected delay in hooking him up for by-pass."

Once the patient was ready in A Theatre, Barnard would give the go-ahead for the donor heart team in B Theatre to switch off Darvall's breathing machine and put her on their by-pass machine. At that point, and that point only, would he go in and remove her heart.

Barnard hurried back to A Theatre to check on progress with Washkansky. Hewitson was cutting a straight line down the centre of the patient's chest. As he cut, he cauterised severed blood vessels. The patient's chest lay open. Peering inside, the surgeon could see the long, flat sternum bone locking together the two sides of the rib-cage like a clamp. But now this lock had to be broken open, like a burglar gaining privileged access to the inner sanctum of the human heart.

Hewitson took up his surgical saw and split the protective breastbone in half, the blades buzzing, wisps of smoke generated by the friction. To stem bleeding from the broken bone, wax was rubbed onto the rough edges. The surgical burglary continued. He was handed a retractor, a hooked steel tool, which he used as a lever to open both gates of the rib-cage and expose the area between the patient's spongy, gray lungs, mottled and tinted dark red.

At this stage, the patient's heart was still out of sight but Hewitson began immediately to cut through the thin, glistening pericardial sac, its web tissue of blood vessels fluttering with the rhythm of blood flow.

At last, Washkansky's weak, but valiant, heart appeared. It seemed almost disorientated, the heartbeat jumping around. It was clearly a diseased organ, discoloured almost to yellow and streaked with scarred tissue and blue veins. It was an organ which had been given a death sentence.

Hewitson's bushy eyebrows lifted and his eyes dilated in sheer disbelief at the sight.

Barnard asked him to show more of the left ventricle. It was a massive, swollen chamber with walls lined with scars. It was a miracle Washkansky was still alive with a heart which had lost so much of the power of its muscles.

"This man will surely only live again if he gets a new heart," Barnard declared, equally bewildered.

Hewitson nodded in agreement. But the two surgeons were hell-bent on giving the patient his new life, giving a new source of power to him. The meaning of the transplant had suddenly been revealed as never before. Hadn't the Old Testament spoken long ago about replacing a lifeless heart with a life-giving one? Now medical science was about to make that happen in a real way. Washkansky's heart was finished, like a wrecked car. But would Denise's heart be strong enough to replace this one?

Barnard instructed his team in A Theatre to get the man lying prone and helpless under the glare of the theatre lights ready for the by-pass machine, that would keep his blood circulating mechanically while his sick heart was cut out.

When he got back into B Theatre, Terry and Marius looked around at him.

"Now?" Marius asked.

Chris looked around, pondering. Everyone looked calm and yet battle-ready. He noted that all the technology and all the surgical instruments seemed to be in place. It was time to turn off Denise's breathing machine.

"Now," his brother confirmed, as Denise Darvall's respirator was turned off.

There was a moment of solemn pause. The donor's breathing had ended. Her brain-dead body would now begin to expire.

The theatre clock read 2.20 a.m.

One by one, the connections to life-supporting tubes and lines were turned off. Death had been let into B Theatre. It would seep through her body. Coert injected blood-thinning Heparin through a drip still tied to her arm. There could be no clotting of her heart arteries.

Barnard was highly focused. He would not let Washkansky go. It was in the bag, wasn't it? He checked Denny's heart monitor. There was no change. The minutes passed. Her heart's pump would not give up.

Dr Venter then closed the taps of the intravenous lines.

"Coert, let's administer some Heparin," Barnard suggested.

Venter already had the solution ready and it began to drip into a tube leading to her inert left arm. It would prevent clotting of her heart arteries.

Already, her lungs were becoming starved of oxygen, draining her blood of its tiny bubbles of life, her blood becoming increasingly toxic. Her heart would begin to feel strangulated, its rhythm disrupted, its muscles struggling to perform their pumping action, like a car engine running out of fuel.

But the donor's machine of life continued to beat, showing its natural vigour. The clock on the wall was now beating faster than her heart was, maintaining its inevitable regularity as Denise Darvall's body began to function ever more erratically.

Marius and Chris Barnard, looking at each other knowingly, watched the minutes pass with some alarm. They were witnessing a good heart collapse, standing by helplessly as the risks to Washkansky increased with each passing second. But Terry O'Donovan refused point-blank to lift a surgical instrument until the ECG flat-lined, indicating the donor's heart had stopped for good. They wanted a flat electroencephalograph. Officially, that would be her moment of actual death. Beyond any shadow of doubt or recrimination.

The Barnard brothers respected his sentiments so the three surgeons simply waited, trapped in suspense. Barnard himself did not want to be perceived as playing God. Yet how could it be considered taking her life when it had already been removed the moment her brain was declared dead and beyond repair? Ah, he reflected as they waited anxiously, the intricacies of medical ethics…

"What do you say, Chris?" Marius enquired.

"No, we must wait until her heart stops."

Five more minutes passed. Tick, tick, tick. Beep-beep-beep. Then another five, each minute becoming interminable in B Theatre.

Then the beats became increasingly erratic, highs followed by the lows of an exhausted organ running out of power. A few moments later, there was a flat green line across the screen signalling her death had finally arrived.

"Now?" Marius asked.

His brother shook his head and held up his hand. Let death finish its work first.

It was just after 2.30 a.m.

The leader of the heart team waited to hear if the heart would start up again. Another minute went by and then yet another.

"Now!" Barnard commanded.

With Denise's life being now officially over, her heart became hospital property. Now it could be removed and used for medical purposes, moving like a queen in a chess game. Terry O'Donovan began cutting.

The lead surgeon dashed into A Theatre. Before heading for the scrub room once more he called out to Hewitson to get the patient hooked onto bypass. The transplant was now imminent.

He always used the same sink on the left. It was a superstitious ritual. While he was lathering up his arms, two important details occurred to him. He went to the door of the theatre, his arms wet with soap.

He shouted to Rodney across the theatre, already teaming with activity, to ask him to insert a catheter into the atrial sac in the muscle wall of the heart's top left chamber. The cool-headed surgeon simply nodded his head. Barnard trusted him implicitly.

"And Ozzie, my man, let's get that Cortisone into his system to kick-start the anti-rejection treatment!"

Ozinsky nodded.

Barnard was about to turn around and head back to finish scrubbing when, trying to control his mounting excitement, he remembered to check that Johan van Heerden was ready to run the by-pass machine.

"Yes, Prof," the pump technician answered.

Although relatively inexperienced, he was already a trusted presence in the theatre.

Barnard went back to the wash-basin. From B Theatre, he heard the searing sounds of O'Donovan's saw cutting through Darvall's chest on his way to exposing her heart for excision.

During the five or so minutes of scrubbing, Barnard kept popping in to each theatre of either side of him, unable to restrain his curiosity.

"Is it all right?" he called out to the surgeons in B Theatre.

"Yes, fine. We've exposed her heart. We're preparing for bypass."

"Is her heart looking alright?" Barnard then asked.

He couldn't resist popping into the theatre to peer into Denise Darvall's exposed interior chest and see her heart, this gift of all gifts. Being used to looking at diseased and bloated hearts in open heart surgery, he was startled to observe what appeared to be a small organ, which, nevertheless, was destined to carry so much responsibility for the success of the operation. It seemed beyond life, inert. The sight shocked him for a moment. Were they too late?

Nervously, he asked Terry what he thought of the blue heart.

"At least we waited for it to stop. I guess it does look rather blue."

Chris was anxious because he knew his parents had lost his older brother, Abraham, to a blue heart at the tender age of two years old. He urged O'Donovan to suffuse the organ with blood by hooking the donor's body to the by-pass pump.

The donor heart was just too blue, too cold, too still for his liking.

With renewed urgency, Marius and O'Donovan connected a catheter from the donor's heart to the machine to suffuse her with living blood. Now that she was deceased in heart and brain, she needed blood circulation from the machine pump. The surgeons also inserted a tube for drainage of any excess blood, which could potentially swell Denise's muscles and cause damage. It was delicate work requiring surgical precision. They all cared so much for the little heart, wanting the best for Washkansky.

"Hurry! Hurry!" insisted the clock on the theatre wall.

As if in response to the call of the clock, Marius instructed the machine to be switched on. He turned to Nic Vermaak and Alastair Hope, who were operating the heart-lung machine in B Theatre.

"Ready, Gentlemen?" he asked them.

Hope was a master pump technician who always did perfect bypasses.

"Ready."

"Pump on!"

Immediately, it was as if Life had been switched back on. The donor's heart, suffused with a flow of blood, turned a fresh pink colour. It firmed up, quivering with a newfound power. But the muscles were not strong enough to pump and there was not yet any heartbeat. Was the heart damaged? The Barnard brothers went ashen-faced as they looked failure in the eye. It seemed they'd waited too long before opening her up to take out her heart.

Perhaps the blood flowing into the deceased donor's heart from the machine was too cold? Barnard wanted to speed up the cooling of her body to help get her heart going again.

He instructed Alastair Hope to cool down the body as fast as possible through the heat exchanger process. He wanted to ensure there would be no cell damage to the muscles of the precious organ, to keep it in the most stable state possible.

Satisfied that the donor was just about ready, the surgeon went back to the scrub room to complete the intensive pre-op cleansing procedure. After getting rid of all dampness, which could incubate germs, he pulled on his favoured thin rubber gloves. The thicker standard ones always aggravated his arthritis. It would be his hands which would be the instruments of peace, of healing and, during surgery, he wanted them to feel as free and manoeuvrable as possible.

A historic time had arrived. This was what he had lived for, trained for, fought for. He was like a fighter getting gloved up who knew he was in tip-top shape.

Barnard stepped confidently into A Theatre. He went to the right side of the operating table after ducking under the line connecting Washkansky to the heart-lung machine. It was time to put the patient on by-pass in preparation for extracting his failing heart.

10

BLOOD ON THE FLOOR

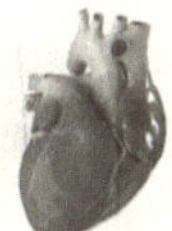

Fourteen members of the heart team were in the theatres to support Barnard in the surgery that lay ahead over the next few hours. Behind them, in the raised amphitheatre so typical of academic hospitals, was an audience of doctors and specialists, also in surgical masks.

Barnard surveyed the scene like a battlefield commander. All eyes hovered on him, waiting for his word. Inside him, all doubt had been cleansed from his mind. The prayer in the shower had seen to that. His heart was ready for action, just as Louis's heart was ready for its salvation. His call to switch on the heart pump rang out in the theatre chamber like a starting pistol at a race or a whistle to begin a highly anticipated match.

The heart-lung machine clicked and whirred into action. Its motors hummed in the expectant silence of A Theatre. Blood pulsed through the tubes, then into the femoral artery, heading for Washkansky's heart until it found its course blocked at the closed aortic valve, whereupon it was diverted into the body to flush its millions of cells. Then, on its return journey through the network of the patient's veins, the blood turned a darker red, almost purple, stained with carbon dioxide waste. The blood flow was heading for the first chamber of the heart, the right atrium, but, once again, was caught by catheters which took it in another direction towards the heart-lung machine. This completed the by-pass circulation: human and machine working as one.

Adrenalin was pumping through Barnard's body, just as blood was coming through the machine's tubes. He checked the pressure of the blood returning into the heart and it was coming down nicely. But there seemed to be nothing stopping the pressure in the lines climbing dangerously high. It was now 240, then 265, then 290. Soon, it would burst open the by-pass lines. What was going on? The ECG beeps punctured the air. Tension rose in A Theatre.

"Line pressure still rising."

Barnard scanned his mind and the scene before him for a possible cause, afraid that the blood would explode out of the machine at such a high pressure. Pieces of medical knowledge and other thoughts flashed through his mind. Somewhere was a blockage of the blood flow – he thought it might be a narrowing of one of the bigger arteries. He stared at the patient's body and noticed, once again, the catheter attached to the groin area. That was it, he thought to himself. It must be the femoral artery that was the culprit. Rodney then confirmed that it did, indeed, look sclerotic, its inside walls packed with plaque build-up. The catheter had to be disconnected immediately. The best move now would be the most direct one: to pass the tube into the aorta itself, the king of arteries!

At that moment, someone kicked a metal bucket and it clanged loudly like a bell in a chamber.

Dene Friedman got a fright and exclaimed. What was even more alarming was the continued increase in the line pressure to 300.

"We've got to stop it there!" Barnard stated, perspiration beaded on his forehead and nose.

"I think it's holding at 300," said Ozzie.

"Johan, don't increase the flow," Barnard commanded. "Cool him down! I want him at 26."

"Yes, Professor."

Now he needed to get the catheter into the aorta. He asked Sister Jordaan for a silk suture, fixed to a needle and clamped in a needle-holder.

Jordaan had worked for Barnard for years as his instrument sister. She could often anticipate what instrument he was going to ask for. There were three trolleys of surgical instruments set out in order. She passed a silk suture to the meticulous surgeon, fixed to a needle and clamped in a needle-holder.

Working rapidly in his efforts to stabilise the patient and to get the bypass functioning properly, Barnard made a circular stitching in the wall of the aorta. As always, his surgical touches were executed slowly, with great care, working finely. After a few painstaking minutes, he stabbed a hole into the centre of the wall so he could plunge the catheter into its flesh. A rubber snare was then slipped over the silk thread and the stitching was tightened. This action caused the aorta's wall to draw around the tube. Now they had a channel fixed securely into it.

Then something inexplicable – and potentially fatal – occurred. Barnard, with uncharacteristic absent-mindedness, gave the wrong instruction.

"Clamp the line," he said, lost in thought for a second or two, his statement not directed to anyone in particular.

Peggy Jordaan, always sensitive to the heart surgeon's requirements and thought processes, immediately assumed this was a directive. So, she clamped it as instructed. Almost at once, this was followed by a blast as the line blew off from its connection to the heat exchanger. Blood poured out onto the floor. Horrified, Barnard realised the machine was still running at full tilt and pressure had risen in the line once it had been clamped. He told Johan and Dene to switch the pump off.

"Is there any air in the machine near the patient?" he gasped.

"Yes, a lot," Johan confirmed.

"Hell, this was one stupid mistake!" Barnard snarled.

When he calmed down, he immediately acknowledged that his own unclear instruction had caused the problem. He disconnected the catheter leading to Washkansky's heart from the pump line. Then he told the pump technician to turn it back on.

Once again, the artificial circulation system started up. Soon, Johan and Dene took hold of hard rubber hammers and began beating the heat exchangers and the tube to knock out the air bubbles stuck in the system. During the process, Ozzie gave encouraging comments to soothe the nerves of the team.

But then Washkansky's heart started to weaken. Barnard glanced worryingly at the erratic patterns on the ECG.

He became annoyed and barked an instruction to Johan to get a move on.

The seconds slipped by. The motors hummed. The ECG beeped. The clock ticked.

"All clear," Johan finally announced, much to the relief of the team.

Barnard then reconnected the line to the catheter and ordered the pump back on as he got the patient's circulation going again.

Again, the patient's dying heart became more erratic.

"The ventricles are fibrillating!" the anaesthetist cried.

Below them, under the glare of the operating lamps, they could see Washkansky's heart faltering, stuttering, as its muscles jerked in spasms of disorder. The sections of his heart were no longer working in unity, his machine of life was packing up before their eyes, which were dilated in shock at seeing the process of death actually at work.

Barnard reflected on what a strong heart it had been, carrying Washkansky through heart attacks and diseases that would have killed a weaker person. But its fight was now ending. It was time to fetch the donor's heart.

But could the tiny heart of the young woman really save the man's life?

When Barnard crossed over into B Theatre to remove Denise Darvall's heart, he was still shaken by the accident of the spilled blood in A Theatre. His confidence had been rocked. The quick recovery had brought some peace back to his soul. But he was not without trepidation as he prepared to cut out the donor's heart. Any wrong incision could ruin the whole operation.

He looked down once more at the little beating heart. He was moved by what he saw, both as a man and as a surgeon. It was a delicately constructed engine of life. And it was a young heart. The transplant would be like youth passing into an older person's body, to breathe fresh life into his being, a vital part of a woman planted into a terminally ill man.

Terry had cleared away some of the fat around the donor's heart to expose it more clearly, in preparation for surgical removal.

"Thank you Terry, that's a great job."

Now that the donor's heart had to be removed, the by-pass was switched off. It was the end of any blood-flow to the donor's body. He left two vents in her heart, one in the aorta, which would be used for infusion of blood when the heart had been transferred to A Theatre, and the other in the left ventricle, which was to function as an outlet for any excess blood or air.

Barnard's hand shook as he took a pair of scissors from Sister Rautenbach. His body was still tense following the error which had almost cost Washkansky his life. His fingers were trembling but he decided to keep working in the belief that his composure would soon return. He worked at a slower pace to instil yet more calm. He took a deep breath as he set about cutting the heart's eight vessels so it could be extracted. He would cut each one as high as possible. Each cut was irreversible – there was no margin for error. Finally, Terry raised the heart so that the four pulmonary veins, two from each lung, could be severed. The small heart was still, like an offering placed on some altar of medicine.

Barnard delicately lifted the heart from the dead woman's body. Marius passed a round metal basin containing ice-cold, salty lactate solution. His older brother placed the heart into the liquid, which covered much of the organ. At the same time, the kidneys were taken out and handed to Dr De Klerk for transportation to Karl Bremer hospital.

His mind was suffused with elation and relief as he began the short walk from B Theatre to A Theatre, carefully balancing the surgical prize, confidence restored after completing the first half of the transplant. He handed the basin to Sister Jordaan at the operating table.

"Don't drop it, Sister, whatever you do!" he told her. It was just after 3 a.m.

She placed the steel container on the theatre towels covering the patient's legs. Denise Darvall's heart was now resting on the body of the man it could save.

"Don't let if fall off!" Jordaan admonished.

Now her heart needed blood: Washkansky's blood. Bosman and Hitchcock hooked up a line from a small perfusion pump, attached to the by-pass machine, to the catheter in the aorta. Blood flowed into the organ like a small stream of life. The joining of her organ to Washkansky's life-giving circulatory system had begun.

The heart surgeon rinsed his cramping hands in a basin. Then he took up his position at the operating table. He surveyed the patient's open chest cavity. He could see the man's heart was quivering, on its last legs, running out of power. But now the donor heart, suffused with blood, had turned a fresher, pinkish colour and Barnard knew he could get on with swapping the hearts. It was time to cut the blood flow to Washkansky's heart. He clamped the aorta below the tube running from the by-pass system. It was the end of the road for a ruined heart.

The surgeon realised he'd entered the second half of the transplant, the last rounds of the fight, and he could sense the procedure was gaining momentum. He noticed that his hands were no longer trembling as he took hold of a small pair of surgical scissors. He was steady, determined there would be no more mistakes that night. Inside his head, he was speaking firmly to himself to reinforce his newfound fearlessness. Take out the heart with more than you need. Get it done, man. You're halfway there.

Barnard made a cut to the aorta. Then he severed the pulmonary artery, which carried blood to the lungs for oxygenation. Its two major vessels cut off, Washkansky's sick heart was almost severed from the body which had hosted it for over five decades.

Its pumping chambers, the ventricles, no longer functioned. But he was about to receive the new machine of a strong, young heart.

Chris's own heart pumped ever stronger, excitement rising up in him with adrenalin to overcome physical and mental fatigue. He sensed that an incredible, dream-like moment was approaching.

11

A NEW HUMAN FRONTIER

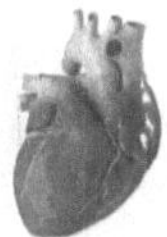

As Professor Barnard cut down through the chambers of the wall of Washkansky's heart, the organ fell back into its fleshy cavity, cut off. It lay still in a shallow pool of blood. The heart surgeon paused, as if frozen, unable to move. As he gazed at the severed organ, he thought of its story, the journey of this man's life, exiled from his birthplace in Lithuania, first to the Crimea and then far from home in Africa's southernmost city. He knew his patient, who'd led a full, varied life, was hungry to go on living.

Barnard reached down and picked up the discoloured and disfigured heart. Then he placed it in a basin held out by Sister Jordaan. Rodney drained and cleaned the pericardium with a pump sucker. The cavity where the heart had been looked like an empty room. A gaping hole was all that was left of Washkansky's chest. A feeling of loneliness enveloped Barnard.

He'd arrived at a threshold of the unknown. There was no one to turn to, to the right, left, front or back, for comforting guidance. From now on, there were no mentors who could answer the questions that would arise. The heart team were on their own, looking to him to lead them home. But he was feeling a little dizzy at the prospect, apprehension having crept back into his bones.

Bossie moved first, handing the basin containing the donor heart to Barnard. The surgeon lifted the little organ into his hands. It was ice cold, apparently lifeless.

Now, he thought back to the idea he'd had while lying on his bed that afternoon in Zeekoevlei. Instead of blindly following the steps of current techniques, which cut away the upper layer of the donor heart so that it could be joined to the lid left behind of the patient's heart, he decided instead to incise the roof of Denise's heart at the points where the veins entered the heart's two upper chambers, intending to stitch these two holes to Washkansky's heart lid later. These two holes could then be stitched to the lid left of Washkansky's heart. Since there were risks associated with the established procedure of cutting into the central wall of the heart's upper chamber, namely that it could harm the organ's conduction system, or cut the coronary sinus, and since the innovation he'd conceived seemed to be comparatively risk-free, he went ahead. As he proceeded, he explained what he was doing to an astonished Rodney Hewitson, saying he'd just conceived of this step that weekend.

It was very late but no one in the theatre, whether participating in the operation or observing it, felt any tiredness. The fact that it was well past midnight added to the sense of the surreal. Under the watchful eye of the clock on the wall, medical history continued unfolding before their eyes.

With these two openings at the top of the donor heart, and two vessels coming from its ventricles, it was ready to be transplanted. With as much care as he could muster, Rodney, the gentleman surgeon, lowered the organ into the gaping space inside Washkansky's chest. Initially, Denise Darvall's heart looked lost inside the patient, given that a woman's heart is much smaller and lighter than a man's. Undeterred, Barnard began sewing the two openings at the top of her heart he'd made, according to the vision he'd seen in his mind, attaching them to what had been left behind of the upper layer of the patient's heart. Like an expert tailor of human flesh, he sewed around the edges and then onto the central septal wall.

Barnard wanted to complete the back part of the heart first. This section would be hardest to reach once the joining had been executed. Here, the suture, or line of sewing, had to be flawless, with no leaks. He stitched first from inside of the heart and then from outside to seal the join. While the two surgeons worked, Bossie and Francois kept the area clean with suckers and retractors. When the suture line was completed, the surgeons inspected it closely.

"Check this for me, there can be no gaps, no faults," Barnard commented.

They strained their eyes as their peered as close to the heart line as they could.

"Over there!" exclaimed Rodney, pointing to a tiny gap in the stitching line on the left side of the atrium.

"That could have killed the man," Barnard said, sewing over the stitching to close it into a tight, continuous line.

After that, the right atrial connection was sewed in the same meticulous way. Six of the smaller vessels had now been connected, part of Denise joined to Washkansky.

Still ahead lay the joining of the two major heart vessels, the pulmonary and aorta. Barnard stitched the pulmonary vessel without any problems. One more step and the donor's heart would belong permanently to the recipient…

Softly, the motors of the heart-lung machine were humming. A catheter was still attached from the by-pass system to Washkansky's hanging aorta vessel, feeding blood into his body. Barnard decided to switch the blood supply off as the aorta artery was swollen with blood and the surgeons needed more space in which to make their final joins.

As soon as the flow of blood stopped, the newly transplanted heart became blue.

It was now 5.15 a.m.

The surgeons took the catheter out of the donor heart because the organ would soon receive living blood from Washkansky. Ozzie circulated warm water through a special rubber mattress to heat up the patient's body.

Barnard cut back the donor's aorta to create a larger opening that would better match the size of the vessel to which it would be joined. The two surgeons began stitching them together.

The delicate and precise process of anastomosis used up priceless minutes and the donor heart went a darker blue, through want of oxygen and blood.

As the theatre clock ticked over to 5.34 a.m., the final suture was sewn. The heart organ had been without any circulation for about twenty minutes. Then the team began to release some blood flow. However, they ran into another danger. There was trapped air bubbling through the suture line in the pulmonary artery.

"Give me the knife!" Barnard instructed. "No air must get into that artery."

Sister Jordaan was struggling to fit a blade.

"Hurry, man!" the surgeon snapped.

Annoyed, the redoubtable theatre sister slapped the handle of the knife into his hand. More air was bubbling out on the stitching. Barnard jabbed a hole into the pulmonary artery and then inserted a sucker to vacuum out the air bubbles. When the newly transplanted heart was free of air, he closed up the hole in the artery he'd made. After that, he released the clamp on the aorta. Then blood was released, passing through the muscles of the woman's heart now inside a man. It tensed and then sprang into life. It began to contract, bursting with new energy. The heart which had last beat inside Denise Darvall three hours before could now pump inside the patient. Would the organ be reborn?

The new heart tensed into action as warm blood flooded its muscles. It began to contract, bursting with new energy.

Barnard immediately thought to himself – her heart wants to live!

"It looks like the heart is becoming more active..." murmured Ozzie, enthralled.

But would the transplanted heart really work, taking over all the functions required of it? Or would it give up, not recognising its new home inside Washkansky? In the animal laboratory, some dogs with newly transplanted hearts had not lived simply because their hearts did not take root inside the foreign organism.

Barnard pondered again on their decision to wait so long for Denny's heart to stop. Would it burst into life again? Certainly, there was not yet any real rhythm to the organ's contractions. The team decided to give the patient electric shocks to help the heart rediscover its natural rhythm.

Ozinsky went to the heart-lung machine and injected 100 mg of Scoline to help the body relax and prevent it from jerking violently when the prescribed voltage was administered.

"All set," Ozzie reported. "Paddles, please."

Barnard grabbed hold of the paddles of the defibrillator to administer the required voltage. He placed the discs on each side of the heart.

"Shock the heart!"

A 20-joules charge of TK volts shot through the muscles, and Washkansky's body arched upwards with the kick of the shock. But the heart remained inert. Moments ticked by. No movement or sign of life. Then, to the amazement of the team members crowded around the operating table, there was a heave of the heart as it began to contract, first the atria, then the ventricles, then the atria, then the ventricles, a regular rhythm building like an engine warming up.

Denise Darvall's heart was beating again.

Inside the open chest, her heart was the star of the show, getting stronger as it contracted, sending out blood on its mission to reach and invigorate the cells of Washkansky's body, and then rolling back. It looked like it had enough power, without help from the heart-lung machine, to push out the blood's circulation.

Rodney and Barnard checked their stitching around the vessels they'd joined. No leaks in the suture lines. No abnormal bleeding. So they prepared to switch off the machine. Barnard removed a vent from the left ventricle and stitched the opening closed. He loosened the tapes around the other catheters in the venae cavae to allow fuller blood flow into the Washkansky's new heart. It took its added load well.

The pump was turned off. Would nature be able to run its course unaided by technology? Dene reported a steady decrease in blood pressure. Unfortunately, the heart began to stumble without machine support. The pressure kept falling, reaching 65. There was no choice but to restart the pump. Barnard told himself that the heart was just getting used to its new surroundings, that it would soon embrace its second life. He asked Ozzie to step up the Isoprenaline dosage to stimulate the heart rate and stabilise blood pressure.

When the by-pass machine was on, the heart functioned well. Now, there was only one catheter left for this mechanical assistance. Washkansky was still part human, part machine.

The bypass system was switched off again, its humming sounds cut out, as a strange silence descended over the theatre. The transplanted heart hesitated, not able, or willing, to jump straight into the pumping action. The blood pressure started to fall.

"By-pass back on!"

The team couldn't seem to get the heart off its apparent dependence on the pump's support.

There were still no leaks along the stitching lines.

"Bossie, the heart doesn't want to work for our poor patient," Barnard reflected, becoming despondent.

This time it was Bosman who kept the fire of belief burning in A Theatre.

"It just wants to be sure it's really alive again," he postulated.

The organ had taken twenty minutes to die, perhaps it would need that amount of time to feel alive?

"Pressure now rising!" exclaimed Ozzie, ever the optimist.

Barnard glanced at the clock: 6.12 a.m. He watched a minute tick by on the timepiece.

"We can do this," he called out. "Turn the by-pass off!"

The motors went off. They watched, eager. There was an aching quiet in the theatre. This time, the heart hesitated for a brief moment and then started pushing and beating with an appetite for life, throbbing with its own energy.

"85 over 60, 80, 90, 90 – it's holding fine Professor – 90, 95,

95!"

Barnard turned in amazement to Johan and Dene, his eyes moist with unrestrained joy.

"Dit gaan werk!"

With these three words of triumph from their leader, spoken from the heart, where a person's mother language lives as part of the soul, confidence flooded into the team and spread to the whole theatre. Everyone sensed the tide was now turning in their favour. Eyes above masks blinked back the tears, there were sighs of wonder, mumbled words, a chuckle of relief, a collective release of tension as thanksgiving filled their drained bodies.

All that remained was to take the patient off by-pass. After the muted celebrations, Barnard looked again at the theatre clock: 6.24.

They had to give back the ability of Washkansky's body to form blood clots so that his multiple surgical wounds could heal. Barnard extracted the last catheter, and completed the stitching up. The transplanted heart was still in perfect control. The ECG showed a steady heartbeat, working in its normal, natural cycles.

In A Theatre of Groote Schuur Hospital, Denise Darvall was doing her customary work of giving, this time from beyond the grave.

Barnard reached out his hand across the open chest where he'd just performed the world's first human heart transplant and took the gloved hand of his assistant surgeon.

"We made it, Rodney."

His part of the operation completed, he left Hewitson to close up Washkansky's chest and walked out of the theatre, removing his surgical gloves, his hands aching, his brain and body numb with fatigue.

He went into the tea room, limp. His brother Marius took his pulse. 140. His colleagues made him a cup of tea to revive him. There was no talk. Outside, another summer's day was slowly beginning in Cape Town.

After a few minutes of rest and reflection, Barnard grabbed his mask and went back to check on his patient.

"He opened his eyes," Ozzie said.

"Good."

"Urine output is good. Brain is fine."

"Great."

Barnard looked at the ECG. The heart was steady, carrying circulation at 120 beats a minute. Boy, did her heart come alive again, the surgeon thought to himself.

After instructing Ozzie to provide the patient with more Cortisone, Barnard returned to the tea room, feeling proud and satisfied.

The anti-rejection treatment was now underway.

"You'd better inform the hospital," Dr M.C. Botha suggested.

Barnard nodded, reaching for the landline to call the medical superintendent.

"Dr Burger?" he said.

"Who's this?" Burger replied.

The hospital's superintendent was a stout, balding white-haired man with a gruff manner.

"Professor Barnard."

"What do you want?"

Burger was a veteran of the life of the hospital, believing he'd seen it all.

"We've just done a heart transplant and thought you should know."

"Your dogs again, Barnard?"

"No, Dr Burger, this time it was humans."

12

A WORLD EVENT

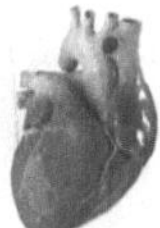

Many unknowns lay ahead. The heart team expected Washkansky's body to fight against the transplanted heart, even though, ironically, it would be attacking the only organ able to keep him alive. The other major threat would be infection.

The world's media was simply asking how long the transplant recipient would live.

A bed was brought into A Theatre for Washkansky to take him to an isolation room. This bed was covered with a sterile plastic tent. Since bacteria would be his main enemy, no precaution was spared. Only personnel and visitors dressed in the protective gear of the operating theatre, including gowns, masks and gloves, would be allowed there.

Barnard's team had prepared a range of immune-suppressive drugs, including Imuran and Hydrocortisone, to fight the body's rejection mechanism.

Of the eighteen lines, tubes and leads connecting the patient to machines, instruments and bottles, nine were now removed, including thermometer leads and ECG electrodes. The remaining nine lines were still needed, essential for feeding the body, relieving waste, monitoring its interior state and administering drugs.

It took six people to lift Washkansky off the table onto this special bed. He was starting to regain consciousness, moving his head from side to side. Then he lifted his arm. The man with the transplanted heart was awakening from his deep, death-like slumber.

"Let's get going," Ozzie urged.

The plastic tent was extended and tucked under the mattress and then the bed was quickly wheeled along the corridor to the elevator. It, too, had been washed down with anti-septic solution. When they got to the sterilised lift, there was not enough room for everyone, so Barnard offered to walk up the one floor to Washkansky's newly prepared isolation ward.

The surgeon returned to the dressing room and changed his clothes. Then he walked up to check on his patient. He was fatigued but had enough adrenalin still in his system to keep him going for a few more hours.

Ozzie had attached a tube from the patient's left nostril to a respirator which was ventilating his lungs at the rate of twenty times a minute. And a gastric tube entering the right nostril was connected to a suction apparatus. Chest drainage lines were joined up to a suction pipe mounted on the wall. In addition, there was a bladder catheter. A venous pressure line was linked to the manometer to measure blood pressure. Electrodes were secured to his upper arms and left leg for ECG monitoring. Finally, there were intravenous drips as part of the life support system.

The donor heart was beating at 110 beats per minute. It was the drumbeat of his new life.

"Let's push up the Potassium," Barnard said, content with the early progress of his patient.

Dr Coert Venter nodded.

The heart surgeon checked the levels of Insulin and Cortisone.

Barnard knew they had to implement, to a 'T', the strict policy of treating the ward like a theatre. Everyone going inside had to scrub and cleanse with the same rigour required before an operation.

He instructed Venter to get the bed washed down and cleansed, including the rollers and the floor.

"No one can enter unless clinically ready," he stated. "Smear Gentamycin ointment on the patient's leg wound and in his nostrils."

Barnard was especially concerned about the infection in Washkansky's left calf.

"Sister, make sure he's kept clean in all parts and watch that dressing in his leg."

"Yes, Professor."

It was at this point that Washkansky opened his eyes. It seemed like he was returning not just from unconsciousness but from death. Delighted to see him coming around, members of the team reassured him he was doing fine. He nodded, and then grimaced, soon drifting off to sleep again.

Shortly afterwards, the heart surgeon noticed some cardiac contractions outside of a normal heart rhythm. There was evidence of some atrial flutter.

"I'll be happier when this settles down," Barnard remarked to Bossie.

"There's a partial heart block," Bosman replied.

"Where are the x-ray people?" Barnard asked, wanting to see the size of the heart and the condition of the lungs.

"They're on their way now."

"Hell, does everything grind to a halt just because it's Sunday?"

Impatient, Barnard left the ward to find Professor Schrire. He wanted to get his evaluation. He always trusted his mentor's wise assessments.

In the corridor, he encountered Ann Washkansky, along with another woman and two men. One of them was Tevia, Louis's brother. The patient's wife stepped forward towards him, a slight smile breaking out nervously on her face.

"How is he, Professor?" she asked in a gentle, concerned voice.

"We are three quarters there. But the final quarter will be hard. We'll fight hard."

"So he has a chance, Doctor?" Tevia asked.

"Yes, he does, if we can hold on to what we have."

"That's good."

"Is he awake?" Ann asked.

"Yes, but he's not yet speaking."

A few awkward moments of silence ensued, the visitors unsure what to do next.

"Please be patient until you can see him, hopefully in a few days."

"Thank you, Doctor Barnard, we understand."

Again, they stood, unsure whether to go or to find out more information.

"I think we need to be grateful for what's happened so far," the surgeon suggested.

"Yes, thank God," Ann replied, reassured.

The visitors then turned around to go, satisfied.

Barnard went into the doctors' office. He called Schrire and asked him to come down for an evaluation of the state of Washkansky's heart. Then he called his wife.

"Louwtjie, ons het geslaag," he told her. "Hy lewe."

"Dit is wonderlik, my skat," she replied, her voice breaking with emotion.

Affirmed by his wife, Barnard suddenly felt a rush of pride in what he and his team had achieved. With a new skip in his step, he went back into the isolation ward.

The x-ray unit had arrived. They produced a picture of the patient's lungs, which were expanded, and of a small-looking heart inside a large cavity.

Meanwhile, the heart rate had dropped and had begun to stabilise at 90. This pleased Schrire when he arrived. The patient opened his eyes for a second time, looking around him.

"You're doing well, Louis," Barnard whispered to him.

There was little bleeding in the chest but, overall, circulation was improving to the periphery of his body. Things were normalising. Everything seemed to be under control, and Barnard decided to return home. Tiredness hit him hard as soon as his intense focus began to dissolve into a more relaxed frame of mind.

He left the hospital with some parting instructions and got into his car. It was almost noon on a lazy Sunday in the Cape.

A few kilometres away, above the city bowl, the noon canon on Signal Hill boomed.

Barnard felt like a different person. The world itself was a changed place.

The 12 o'clock news was being broadcast on the car radio as he drove back towards Zeekoevlei.

"The first human-to-human heart transplant in history was done last night by a team of doctors at Groote Schuur Hospital. The names of the patient and donor are being withheld by hospital authorities…"

The glare of sunlight was brilliant all around him and he felt the need to get home and rest because he was struggling to keep his eyes open behind the wheel of his car. He was drowsy with exhaustion. Frankie Valli's catchy single "Can't Take My Eyes Off You" on the radio cheered and energised him. When he turned into his driveway in Flamingo Crescent, Louwtjie ran up to meet her husband. Her eyes glistened with excitement as she hugged him.

Suddenly, he was just a man again, not a path-finding surgeon.

"I phoned Deirdre to tell her," Louwtjie said.

"And Boetie? Did you tell him?"

"I placed a call but haven't got through yet."

Inside the home, things were the same as always, yet not the same, because the phone began to ring from all corners of the world. The first call was from a newspaper in Fleet Street.

"Did you really transplant a human heart?" the reporter asked.

"Yes, we did."

"Was it a white heart…that is, from a white person?"

"It was a strong heart," Barnard replied.

"Was the patient Jewish?"

"What's that got to do with it?"

"Is his name Louis Washkansky?"

"How do you know that?"

"It's in the news bulletin."

"Yes, then, it was Mr Washkansky."

How long would it be before the media would dig up the name of the donor, too?

"What sort of man is Mr Washkansky?"

"He's a man with a new heart," Barnard answered.

After the interview with the newspaper in London, calls came from reporters and well-wishers from several countries.

Later in the afternoon, Barnard called the hospital. He was informed that Washkansky's pulse rate had gone from 90, which is what it was when he'd left Groote Schuur, to 120 and then even further up to 140.

"The urine output has diminished to 50, but everything else seems alright," said Coert Venter.

"I'm coming in," Barnard replied, unable to sleep or rest.

"Shouldn't you rest, skat?" Louwtjie asked.

"When he's okay," her husband replied.

Barnard got into this car and headed back to the hospital. By the time he'd reached Washkansky's ward on his return, about half an hour later, the patient's pulse rate had returned to 85. Reassured, he made a few adjustments to the treatment and then went home again, this time resolving to get some real sleep. He simply couldn't keep going any longer.

He slept deeply that night but awoke early the next day, his brain teeming with thoughts and imagined scenarios. Would Washkansky speak on his first full day after the invasive trauma of open-heart surgery? What would his vital indicators show? Had he gone downhill overnight?

Barnard called the hospital first thing. Sister Papendieck answered, her night duty ending.

"How's our patient?" he asked her.

"He looks pink, with a healthy glow," she answered.

These words sounded like a melody to him, causing him to smile, pride once again welling up inside him.

Christiaan then double-checked that there were no signs of anything going wrong and told her he would come over.

Although his body was still tired, and his hands ached, he was in high spirits as he drove through the southern suburbs, past the ivy-covered buildings of the University of Cape Town on the slopes of the mountain, towards Groote Schuur. It was milder than the weather had been at the weekend, with a blustery south-easter cooling the air.

When he arrived at the cardiac unit, Dr Bosman met him in the corridor. He had a big smile on his face. This spoke volumes.

"Dit gaan goed met hom," Bossie confirmed.

Excited, Barnard scrubbed and then dressed in his surgical outfit. He was like a small boy about to open his Christmas presents. When his patient looked up, Barnard noticed his face had softened, no longer grimacing in pain and discomfort.

He greeted Louis.

"I hear you're doing fine," the surgeon said.

Washkansky nodded. He motioned to Barnard for the tube to be removed from his windpipe so he could say something. He was desperate just to say something. Is not speech the voice of the beating heart?

Just let me talk so the world will know I'm still here. I want to re-connect to humanity, to communicate with others, just as much as I want to breathe.

"Hang on, I'll see what I can do," Barnard replied.

The patient dozed back off to sleep. The surgeon waited for Ozinsky to arrive, which happened at about 9 a.m.

"Let's put him in an oxygen tent," Ozzie suggested, "before we disconnect the respirator."

"Agreed, we can see if he can breathe for himself before we take out the tube."

They saw that Washkanksy was breathing well under these conditions so after an hour and a half, Ozzie removed the tube.

Barnard asked his patient how he was doing.

"I'm feeling fine," the reborn man in the oxygen tent replied.

For Washkansky, at that moment, just talking seemed like a small personal triumph, a priceless luxury. He was living again. Barnard had believed all along that such a feat was possible. He'd planned meticulously for years to realise that goal. Even so, it was still amazing to actually talk to someone hosting a heart which had originally belonged to someone else.

"Do you know what we've done?" the surgeon asked, his eyes twinkling.

"Did you really give me the heart you promised?" Washkansky asked.

"Yes, we did. It's beating beautifully."

Washkansky smiled softly, content. This was why Barnard loved medicine: when he could see relief on the faces of his patients. He was helping God's greatest creation – the human body - to work better so that people could improve their well-being and restart their lives. This all gave him an incredible sense of power: an indisputably benign power. From his days at the anatomy laboratory at UCT's medical school, where, using Gray's Anatomy, the Body Bible for medical students, he'd dissected corpses to understand how the body works, to his time in America working under Dr Wangensteen, he'd accumulated his knowledge and skills with a savage relish.

Returning the smile, the heart surgeon explained to the patient that he'd be moved every two hours to help clear his lungs and stimulate his breathing. He also told him the nursing staff would be taking blood samples and giving medicines.

"Try to sleep as much as possible in-between these disturbances," Barnard advised.

The heart surgeon wondered how long it would be before the patient asked whose heart he'd been given. But he didn't ask. Instead, he just gave Barnard a "thumbs up" gesture. Here was a man who had always given life his all – and this time of convalescence would be no different.

Denise Darvall would have been happy to see him smiling.

13

NEW HEART

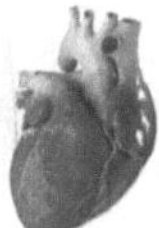

In the days following the heart transplant, Groote Schuur Hospital was besieged by representatives of the international media. Some reporters even masqueraded as doctors and orderlies to try to get access to Washkansky's isolation ward. A few photographers climbed trees outside the window to get shots. Although the heart team began giving regular press conferences, the hunger for news and images about the event, and its aftermath, was insatiable. Meanwhile, telegrams and letters poured in from around the world. For a while, Barnard enjoyed all the attention.

Then, on the Monday afternoon after the operation, Washkansky's condition worsened. His venous pressure had risen and the blood urea was up. Enzymes had increased, too, indicating potential cell damage. This was the first setback.

Barnard thought the transplanted heart might be damming blood back instead of pumping it forward. That would've explained the poor circulation to the kidneys evident in the readings. If the donor heart did not mesh with the recipient's circulatory system, the host body would reject the organ. This was the heart surgeon's biggest fear.

He decided to draw on the additional expertise of a wide range of specialists at Groote Schuur. In the days after the operation, he turned the doctors' office of C2 ward into Mission Control, holding daily meetings. From there, Barnard was focused on masterminding the recovery process.

First, he called Dr Geoffrey Thatcher, a well-respected nephrologist who could help him monitor the functioning of the patient's kidneys and the regulation of blood pressure. Then he phoned Professor Lennox Eales, head of the hospital's renal unit, and biochemists Dr Gideon Potgieter and Professor James Kench. He also appealed to the services of Dr Simcha Banks and Dr Arderne Forder, bacteriologists, as well as Dr Leslie Werbeloff, a radiologist. Above all, of course, he would depend on Professor Schrire as the hospital's most senior cardiologist. Together, they would all combat the twin threats of rejection and infection.

Washkansky himself was all smiles when the surgeon went on his morning round on Tuesday, the second full day after the operation.

"Good morning," the patient said, cheerfully.

"Good morning, Louis, how are you?"

"Very fine. I think."

"Don't you know?"

"Hell, Doc, they never leave me in peace long enough to know how I feel!"

Barnard turned to Sister Georgie Hall, a smile breaking inside his mask.

"Now, Sister Hall, what are you doing to this poor man?"

"Nothing at all, Professor, we love him dearly."

Washkansky shook his head in disagreement.

"They keep rolling me back and forth. It's like trying to sleep on a boat in a storm!"

Sister Hall laughed.

"Doc, this is worse than a boxing match. I get no rest in between rounds!"

"Sister, please treat Mr Washkansky with some Tender Loving Care!"

"Tender Loving Care? Every time I close my eyes they sneak up on me and stick another needle into me. This is a really dangerous place. I hope you're going to give me danger pay."

Barnard was delighted that Washkansky was back, the man who was the tease, the joker, the party man.

When Dr Bosman came in soon afterwards, the patient closed his eyes in mock exasperation.

"Here comes Dracula!" he quipped.

Laughter echoed through the ward.

Afterwards, Barnard went to his first multi-disciplinary meeting along the corridor in the doctors' office. The patient's heart was functioning well so it was a very positive meeting. Each of the specialists the heart surgeon had convened gave a different perspective on Washkansky's complex and nuanced physiological condition.

Biochemist Dr Potgieter had found good and bad signs in the blood samples. On the positive side, the haemoglobin had gone up, revealing more red cells in the blood. The cells carrying the anti-bodies which could cause rejection of an organ, the lymphocytes, had greatly decreased as a result of the immune-suppressive drugs.

On the negative side, Pottie, as he was known by his colleagues, had found that the blood urea had gone up from 82 to 105. This indicated a level of toxicity which wouldn't have been there if Washkansky's kidneys were functioning normally.

"We have to take into account the damage done by the surgery itself," Barnard argued. "This count should drop."

"It's too early to say from one day's reporting," cautioned Professor Eales, frowning as if to emphasise his point.

But everyone in the room knew they were dealing with something unprecedented, a medical first. If they made judgements based only on past research and experience, they might end up making serious mistakes. They were on a new path.

The team concluded that there was not yet sufficient evidence to support either the rejection or the infection approaches to recovery. They reviewed the current anti-rejection treatment. The plan was to reduce the first massive dose of 500 mgs of Hydrocortisone, given on the day of the operation, by 100 mgs each day until it was stopped altogether. After that, it would be replaced by Prednisone, another corticosteroid. They were also injecting 150 mgs of Imuran each day to protect all the surgical incision wounds from infection.

It was decided to give the patient some radio therapy to destroy the lymphocytes invading the heart.

Later that day, the patient's appetite improved. He was able to enjoy a bowl of soup and a soft-boiled egg.

On Wednesday, the third day of his convalescence, Washkansky was still in good spirits. When Barnard scrubbed up and entered the ward, he heard Sister Hall laughing again.

"I'm the new Frankenstein," the patient declared. "I'm going to scare people off the streets."

"You're more like an angel than a Frankenstein," Sister Hall replied, stoking the patient's ego.

"Are they still giving you acupuncture, Louis?" Barnard enquired.

"I'm a human pin cushion!" the patient quipped. "I can tell you, Doc, they're taken more blood from me than is going back in!"

Professor Schrire, who was there checking on the heart signs, smiled at the repartee.

"The atrial flutter is unimportant at this stage, Chris," he explained. "The heart's in a good condition, beating marvellously. His murmur has disappeared. There's no enlargement of the liver. Don't worry – he's clinically well."

When Barnard told the doctors at their meeting that Washkansky thought he was now Frankenstein, he was corrected. It was the doctor who created the monster who was called Frankenstein in Mary Shelley's Gothic novel, he was told.

"So I'm Doctor Frankenstein," Barnard announced, causing jocularity in the room as he acted out the part.

The signs of progress had encouraged everyone.

However, Dr Bernard Pimstone, who was treating Washkansky's diabetes, reported that the patient needed a much bigger calorie intake.

"This guy needs lots of calories to recover," he explained. "And pump lots of glucose in his cells through the insulin. Otherwise, he's going to start burning too much of the basic proteins of his own body."

"What do you suggest, Bernard?"

"Give him steak, whatever he feels like. He really needs more energy."

Afterwards, as a result of this advice, the patient's diet was increased to include minced chicken and mashed potatoes. It was encouraging for theatre staff to see Washkansky eating this food with relish.

Each day, approaches from the world's media, special correspondents, reporters and television crews, continued almost without interruption.

Despite the signs of recovery, deep down, Barnard felt unsettled. Washkansky was progressing well - but not as well as the surgeon would've wanted. That night, around midnight, he phoned from home to check on the patient's pulse rate. It had risen to 140. The temperature, however, was normal.

Barnard fell asleep telling himself his patient's heart rate would surely settle down during the night.

The next morning, on the fourth day after the operation, the heart rate increased further to 150 and there was persistent atrial flutter. Yet Washkansky had slept well, enjoyed a good breakfast and had no temperature.

The only worry was that Denise Darvall's heart was still refusing to settle down inside his chest.

"When do you think I can go home, Doc?" Washkansky asked when Barnard went into his ward.

"If your recovery continues, not too long," the surgeon replied, hiding his nagging doubts about the erratic performance of the donated heart.

"Will I be home for Christmas?"

"Christmas?" Barnard asked, calculating in his mind how many days were left until the big public holiday.

"Perhaps, let's just wait and see."

"I'll be home for Christmas….Good old Bing Crosby."

Barnard noticed the pulse had improved by falling to 144.

But at 2.30 p.m. the pulse rate rose again to 150, then to 160. Worried, Barnard called Schrire who came immediately to see what was happening.

"This isn't good," the senior cardiologist said, "we must slow down the heart rate."

"With what?"

"Digoxin."

Barnard objected that Shumway and Lower had found that transplanted hearts were sensitive to Digoxin.

"But that was with dogs, this is a human," replied Schrire.

"I'd prefer to go with Strophanthin, which acts for a shorter time than Digoxin," Barnard decided.

"Okay, let's do it your way," Schrire agreed.

That afternoon, Ann Washkansky was allowed to visit her husband for the first time since the operation. She was nervous, not knowing what to expect. The scrubbing and cleansing procedure, followed by dressing in rubber gloves, cap, green gown and washable overshoes, made her feel even more awkward. Besides, who would she be seeing, her husband or a total stranger, a man with a woman's heart?

Her husband was lying flat on his back when she approached the bed.

"Louis, it's me," she said, tentatively.

"Hello, Kid," he replied, a smile edging out across his face.

Instantly, she knew it was the old Louis she loved, not some stranger. He'd always called her "Kid". She was elated.

"You can stand closer," Sister Georgie Hall urged. "But no touching please."

Ann was afraid she would infect her husband.

"Ah, you mean no kissing then, Sister?" Washkansky retorted.

"How do you feel, Love?" Ann asked.

"On the top of the world," he responded. "I've got it under control."

"I knew you'd pull through," she said. "Hey, do you know you're world famous?"

"You're kidding!"

"No, your name is running on the top of Sanlam Building in the city."

"Serious?"

"Everybody's talking about you."

"It's the doctor who should be famous, not me."

"You were incredibly brave, Love."

"I took a chance in my favour, a gambling man to the end," Washkanksy answered.

"You always said you'd be famous," Ann remarked.

Washkansky winked at his wife and she wanted to touch him and to hold him again, feeling she was hiding something from him, behind the surgical mask. Emotions began to well up in her heart. Yet, she could only stand there helplessly, trying to be brave.

Sister Hall told her gently that she had to leave. The timing was perfect because she was about to burst into tears.

"Goodbye, Kid. Don't start any of your old tricks now until I get back home to look after you," he said, looking up at his wife.

"Oh, Louis, I'm so happy I could cry…"

"No, please don't do that…I'm not strong enough yet."

"Goodbye, Louis."

"Goodbye."

Outside, she was asked by a reporter how her husband looked.

"Beautiful," she replied.

14

DAYS OF A MIRACLE

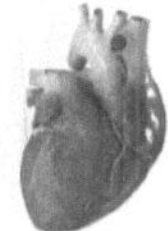

As Barnard drove to the hospital on Friday, 8th December, his main issue was still the potential for Washkansky's body to reject the transplanted heart. A news bulletin flashed over the radio: Louis Washkansky's body may start to reject the donor heart he received, Professor Jannie Louw, chief of Surgery at Groote Schuur, has stated. In a radio interview from his bedside, the most famous patient in the world described the heart surgeon as the man with golden hands.

Barnard looked at his hands on the steering wheel. There was nothing golden about them. Each day, he scanned his hands for any signs of an encroaching arthritic deformity. It pained him when strength seemed to leave them, rendering even simple surgical procedures difficult to perform.

When he arrived at Washkansky's ward, he found his patient equally deflated.

Louis asked to be left alone.

"What's wrong?"

The patient complained of being continuously disturbed. He was tired of being prodded, poked, monitored and tested. Here was a human being feeling trapped in his own body, wanting to break free. Barnard, moved, promised him he would provide some relief. He'd heard the cry of Louis's heart.

Dr Bosman, looking concerned, arrived with a cardiograph print out. It showed a drop in the heart voltage. As a blood pump, the heart had its own power source, an electrical control system in a bundle of nerve fibres in the sinoatrial node. Its regular impulses enabled the organ to contract its muscles. Barnard wondered why his patient's voltage had dropped. Was this, perhaps, the beginning of the rejection process?

Washkansky's pulse rate had risen, once again, to 150. In addition, he was in a weakened state of mind and had become uncharacteristically irritable.

Did trouble lie ahead that day?

"I tell you what, Louis, we'll arrange for you not to be disturbed so you can get some sleep. How does that sound?"

"Thanks," he murmured, his mind and body nearing the limit of their endurance.

Barnard and Bosman felt sorry for him. They decided rest was needed most so at 9.30 a.m. they injected 20 mgs of Pethadine and the patient went straight into a deep sleep. When Washkansky woke up after a few hours' sleep, he was refreshed and in better spirits. He had a good appetite, too.

But the day seemed determined to be a bad one. In the afternoon, his heart voltage sank even further. The team was aware of the link Shumway and Lower had established between decreases in voltage and organ rejection. Barnard concluded that they would lose their patient if they did not start full anti-rejection treatment.

They continued the Imuran dosage but increased the Prednisone to 200 mgs a day. They also decided to give 200 mgs per day of Actinomycin C for a period of three days. Dr Simcha Banks warned them that such a high dose of steroids could lead to acute stomach ulceration with internal bleeding. The bacteriologist recommended the counter-measure of alkalis administered to neutralise these acids.

"Bossie, tell the nurses to be vigilant about the anti-acids and to do bedside tests for sugar in the urine," Barnard instructed.

This was not all the bad news for the day.

"I've found a dangerous pathogen in the patient's system," reported Dr Forder, the bacteriologist. "Klebsiella. I found one in his left nostril, his mouth and in a rectal swab."

This information, coming on top of the other bad signs, froze Barnard's blood and bones.

O, God, things have taken a turn for the worse.

"Klebsiella can cause a wide range of disease states, notably pneumonia, septicaemia and urinary tract infections," Forder explained.

"I suggest we stop using Tetracycline as an antibiotic because it increases vulnerability to fungal invasions," Dr Thatcher recommended.

"What do you suggest, Geoff?"

Thatcher recommended a dose of Gentamycin.

Rejection. Infection. They were fighting a war on two fronts. In fighting one – rejection - they'd leave the patient open to attack from the other - infection.

"We can't lose this man," Barnard insisted, his voice trembling.

Then it happened. Another miracle. Unexpectedly, Louis Washkansky woke up full of life, bursting with spirit, empowered by the mysterious wonder of being alive, as if an electric charger had been plugged into him, or a light switch had been turned back on in his mind.

"Sister Papendieck, when can we take off this candy wrapping?" he asked, referring to the plastic oxygen tent covering him.

She smiled broadly, sensing the old, chirpy Washkansky had returned.

"I guess that makes you the sweet something under the wrapping, Mr Washkansky?"

The patient grinned.

"And you can take this drip off, I'm ready for some real food. How about steak and eggs?"

When Barnard arrived, he could see there was a new happiness radiating from the man who wanted to live life to the full: nothing less was good enough for him.

Washkansky's signs had all improved so the tent was removed, along with the last drip line. His transplanted heart had steadied. All that was still connecting him to machinery were the electrodes on his chest running to the ECG monitor. It was a liberating moment for everyone.

He was given a radio, which had been sterilised, and he began to re-connect to the outside world for the first time since the operation. He listened to news bulletins about himself and to his favourite stations. One report speculated that he might begin to reject the heart of Denise Darvall.

"If they think I'm giving up this heart, they can forget it," he declared. "I never felt better in my life…or happier."

Happier…happiness. You needed a heartbeat for that. You needed the pulse and flow of blood through you to feel good. You needed the electric pulses driving the heart to feel strong. You needed to feel hunger, strength and desires to recover a will to live.

"Hey, Sister," he joked, "do you think I'll grow breasts like a woman?"

Sister Georgie Hall, now on duty in place of Papendieck, smiled, blushing.

"You? Never!"

Softly in the background, Washkansky's radio was playing "Girl, You'll Be a Woman Soon" by Neil Diamond. Barnard thought about Denise and how harsh it had been that her life had been cut short before she'd reached her prime. It made him feel sad for Edward Darvall, too. Yet, his brave decision to allow his daughter's heart to be donated had already been vindicated in full.

A day or two later, during this upbeat period of recuperation, the surgeon quizzed Washkansky on what he was thinking when he regained consciousness after the operation.

"I woke up and I knew something was different," he replied. "I didn't know what. Then I realised, I can breathe. I was breathing, not gasping for air. My heart had been fixed up and I could breathe normally."

It was the first time Washkanksy had called the organ his heart. After all, it was living inside his body, stitched to his own circulatory system, pumping his blood. It was part of his life now, a key to his future.

Scenes from his life passed before his mind's eye as he mused on the path of his destiny, thinking all the time how fortunate he was just to be alive, his death bed left behind him. He was expecting to walk out of the hospital soon.

Having got so close to death, he couldn't get enough of thinking about life and enjoying all its simple pleasures. He came alive so beautifully in those days. When his sister, also called Ann, came to see him, they reminisced together about their early life in Lithuania.

They'd lived in Slabodka, the Jewish part of Kovna. Washkanksy had been the youngest of four children, two boys and two girls. Often, while his mother had worked late in the store they owned, his granny and older sisters had told the little boy stories. But when he was only three, the First World War had broken out.

It was then that the Russians came into Slabodka, accusing Jewish people of being spies for the Germans. Gradually, the intimidation escalated. At one point, the invaders gave Jews there twenty-four hours to leave their homes. Refugees were then packed into trains like cattle. The fleeing Washkansky family had travelled for seven days and seven nights, arriving in the end at Meletrople, next to the Black Sea, in the Crimea. His mother started selling goods at a market near the port to earn a living: socks, shoelaces and stockings. During the next four years there was trouble and fighting between communist forces and white Russians, with no stable government. Sometimes their shop was raided, the family hiding under their beds. There was no enduring safety so they'd decided to return to Slabodka.

That journey back home, riding on cattle cars, had taken two months. They'd carried with them some scarce articles for barter with officials, like candles, soap and flour. But when they got back they found their home was deserted, its roof in a state of collapse.

It was during those years of danger and exile that Louis Washkansky had learnt how tough the world is and how tough you needed to be in order to survive. A fighter had been born. When he was nine years old, his family had emigrated to South Africa, where they'd lived in the Gardens area of the city bowl.

Slowly, gradually, Denise Darvall's heart settled into its new home. It took over all the functions of the heart. Her legacy seemed to be intact. Now, Washkansky's kidneys and liver could once more draw fresh blood through this renewed circulation and the blood could do its daily healing, cleansing, invigorating work.

With his improved blood flow, the wound festering in the patient's left calf began to heal. New blood meant new life and vitality. Louis had been restored in full - to the delight of family, friends and hospital staff.

"Well if it isn't Father Christmas," he said to his brother-in-law, Solly Sklar, dressed in hospital gowns, during a visit.

"Speaking of which, perhaps we can even get him home by Christmas," Barnard remarked. "I'm sure you can make it, Louis."

Noting that Washkansky was in high spirits, Solly promised to organise a welcome home party.

"How's your leg?" Barnard asked Washkansky.

"Look - like new!" the patient replied.

On the Saturday afternoon before the operation, the leg had been badly swollen with the infected sore and his foot had turned blue. The limb had gone cold, with no life in it, no blood-flow. Now, it was a healthy, natural colour.

Seeing Washkansky getting stronger, Solly smiled to himself, thinking back to when he'd met him. In those days he'd been known as Washy. The two men were in their late twenties and were without a care in the world. As a young man, Washkansky had developed a strong frame and body, working out at the Maccabi Wrestling Club and Gym, keen on weight-lifting and wrestling. They'd become friends when they'd discovered they were both from Lithuania. Then, when the Second World War broke out, they'd joined the South African Engineers and had fought in Italy.

"Hey Washy, remember when you made that contraption in the war to brew beer from raisins and orange skins!" Solly said.

"It was my own little chemistry experiment," Washkansky mused. "But I traded that beer for lots of goodies – fresh eggs and even fresh meat. Remember?"

Solly thought to himself how popular Washkansky had been among the troops. A heart of gold man. He also remembered how his friend had refused to wear the standard issue army boots – and then had charged the defence force for the wear and tear to his own footwear.

Only six months after the end of the war, Washy had married Solly's sister, with whom he'd fallen madly in love.

The second time Solly visited his brother-in-law in the ward, on the tenth day, he was astounded to see his mate doing some exercises with a physiotherapist.

"Hey, Solly, I'm going to be running right out of here at this rate!"

Washkansky's stitches hurt him a little during the exercises but he seemed to be getting stronger every day. The wires from his chest to the heart monitor were removed. Now he could move freely. He was becoming a whole man again. He was free.

That day, the two friends spoke about the future, not the past, their conversation spiced with hope.

"I'll get out of here soon," Washy vowed. "Then you and I can go back to Italy and see how the old place looks now."

"We can check out if any of the bridges we built there are still standing," Solly agreed.

"Israel, Solly, we should go there, too. All of us together. A kind of pilgrimage."

"Yes, Louis. Next year in Jerusalem, as they say."

"But, you know what? Even if we never get to Jerusalem, it's been wonderful."

"What has?"

"Just to live again, man. To breathe again. To talk again. Just to have this gift, this time to breathe and to think, is enough, you know what I mean?"

When a photographer came into the ward, Solly excused himself.

He was never to see his friend look so perky again.

134

15

____

SHADOWS APPEAR

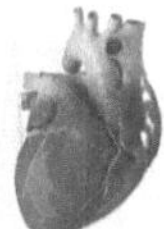

On the Wednesday night, during the second week of recovery, Washkansky woke up three times with severe abdominal pains. He was given snacks and milk to stave off the hunger pangs. After eating, the patient slept soundly.

The staff were trying to neutralise with alkalis any excess acid secretions in the stomach resulting from the intake of steroids. The last thing the patient needed was an ulcer.

At 6 a.m. Louis awoke, feeling tired and irritable. After a good breakfast, he felt better.

He was expecting visits from his Rabbi, the mayor of Cape Town, Gerry Ferry, and an overseas television crew.

Suddenly, a single thought made Washy perk up.

"Sister, I'm getting lots of visitors today so I think I'll shave myself."

The nurse sat him up in his bed and then handed him his shaving kit.

"A man's a nobody if he can't shave himself," he mused, squinting into the mirror and twisting his mouth as he began shaving.

Sister Papendieck followed his every move, fascinated and delighted. She, too, longed for Louis to live fully again.

When the patient finished shaving, he looked proudly at himself in the mirror.

"Hmmm, that felt so good," Washkansky muttered, looking at himself in the mirror with renewed pride, as he stroked his chin and felt his smooth face.

"You look handsome, I must say."

"So, you mean you'll come to my homecoming party, Sister?"

"Wouldn't miss it for the world."

"May I ask you for a dance?"

"It's a date, Mr Washkansky," Sister Papendieck answered, smiling behind her mask.

Suddenly, Louis became serious.

"You know, I'll never have words to thank Professor Barnard for what he's done for me."

Later, the expected visitors started to arrive and it turned out to be a tiring day. Firstly, Rabbi Israel Abrahams appeared, along with Washkansky's brother, Tevia.

The Rabbi reminisced about officiating at Louis's wedding in the Gardens Synagogue two decades previously. He recalled how much the couple had been in love.

"We're still in love 21 years later," Washkansky mused.

The next visitor was the Mayor of Cape Town, an acquaintance from the patient's youth. He, too, spoke about the old days.

"What should I tell the people of the Mother City from its famous son?" Ferry asked, before he left.

"Just say Louis says: 'Merry Christmas and a Happy New Year, Cape Town.'"

By the time some family visitors came to see him, his strength had waned. The visitors included his son Michael, Gracie Sklar, his sister-in-law, and his niece, Chavia Taibel.

On another floor of the hospital, Washkansky's brother-in-law, Daniel Taibel, a Russian Jew whose family had come to South Africa to escape persecution, happened to be dying of cancer. The two men had been closer than brothers for years. Every Sunday, they would eat bagels and Jewish polony together, washed down with some schnapps.

The two men had become ill about the same time, Louis with heart trouble and Daniel with cancer. So when Washkansky saw Chavia, he had only one question on his mind.

"How's Daniel?"

"Daddy's upstairs," was all she could say, turning to Gracie.

"How's Daniel?" he asked his sister-in-law, deeply concerned.

"Like Chavia says, he's upstairs, hanging on, holding on."

Washkansky could read between the lines and he became sad, tears welling up in his eyes. Conversation petered out. After a short spell of sobbing, he looked exhausted. He asked his visitors to leave.

"Get some rest, Louis." Gracie said.

That night, Washkansky once again woke up three times, complaining of stomach pains. He was given milk and toast, as well as antacid pills.

Another night of disturbances left him in low spirits the following morning. He complained of feeling tired. Yet his new heart was performing very well. When he heard his wife had recovered from a cold and sore throat and would be able to visit him later, he cheered up.

But then the BBC managed to disturb his equanimity. An interview had been agreed to, so Washkansky was given a sterilised phone, set up by a local telephone company. At 3.00 p.m. the call came through from the BBC studios in London. "Congratulations on being so famous," they told the patient.

"No, it's the doctors who are famous, not me."

A brief conversation followed.

The reporter asked him how he felt as a man to have a female heart.

"As long as it's a good heart, that's all that matters," he replied.

The interview then became even more personal after that. They asked him how he experienced having the heart of a Gentile. Washkansky became uncomfortable.

"I don't know," he stammered, caught off guard, "I haven't really thought about it."

At this point, an incensed Dr Bosman ordered the interview to be cut.

Outside, sound technicians of the BBC apologised on behalf of their organisation for the offensive question. After that, a CBS crew arrived from America to interview Washkansky. When they left, he was ashen with fatigue.

His wife Ann mentioned that she thought he was getting a cold.

"No way, dear, just tired."

"I think he might have a cold, Sister," she said to Georgie Hall.

"If you want me to have a cold, Kid, then I'll have a cold!" Louis retorted in mock exasperation.

"Listen to him, he's not even home yet and he's already getting out of control!" Ann responded. "What am I to do with my husband, Sister Hall?"

"It looks like you're going to have to cuff him," the nurse exclaimed, hands on her hips.

Ann began to get tearful.

"You don't have to cry about it," Washkansky said.

"I'm sorry, Louis, I just can't help it."

"I told you I have it in the bag, remember?"

"If you tell me then I believe it is so," his wife answered, getting ready to leave.

"You'll come tomorrow?"

"Yes, I'll be here."

"Take it easy and don't get another cold."

"No, I promise I won't…goodbye."

"Goodbye."

Meanwhile, Barnard was still being besieged by reporters and photographers down at the nearby medical school. The telephone in his office was also inundated with calls from newspapers, magazines and even other doctors, many of them foreign.

Just before he was about to go home, his mind crowded with thoughts and echoes of statements and questions from these numerous conversations with the mass media, he received a call from Dr Bosman, urging him to stop by Washkansky's ward on his way out.

"Why, what is it?" Barnard asked.

"Something you should look at in Washkansky's x-ray. There's a part I don't understand."

"What is it, man? Speak clearly, spell it out."

"A shadow has appeared on his lung."

A feeling of dread came over the heart surgeon. What was it now?

"I'm really not sure, it's very tiny," Bossie explained, "but I want you to have a look."

Barnard told himself there was nothing to worry about. Had they not dealt with so many complications already, worries which had turned out in the end to be minor, rather than life-threatening?

"Okay, I'll be there rightaway," he said, overcoming his fear, for the moment, that something new and sinister was amiss.

As he left the medical school to drive up the hill to the hospital, he was confronted by members of the media.

Annoyed, he was brusque with them as he got into his car and pulled away, wishing to be alone so he could think about this patient and plan the next phase of his treatment.

At Groote Schuur, he ran up the stairs to ward C-2. Bosman came out of Washkansky's ward clutching the latest x-ray which the two men discussed in the doctors' office.

"Show me where the shadow is," Barnard asked.

"There," Bossie said, pointing to a small dark grey area he'd spotted on the left lobe of the lung.

Barnard held the x-ray up to the light.

"Hmmm…" He murmured.

"He says he doesn't feel well," Bosman said.

"His temperature is a bit high."

Then they compared the x-ray to the previous one. The difference between them was not significant.

"The patient is seeing too many people," Barnard said, "He needs more rest."

"I agree."

Later, while driving home to Zeekoevlei, Barnard was unable to shake off all the uncertainty about his patient's condition which had now entered his mind. However, he still believed the operation had been a success and that his patient would recover.

The next day was the 13th day of recuperation following the heart transplant. Christmas was just over a week away. Would Louis's dream of being home for Christmas come true?

But the patient was struggling with his breathing, which had become low-pitched and sticky, indicating some fluid in the lungs, some consolidation of lung tissue. As the tissue became filled with liquid, rather than being aerated with gas, it swelled and hardened. It was this consolidated tissue which had shown up on the latest x-rays, being more radio-opaque than aerated lung tissue normally looks.

The medical team now knew for sure that Washkansky's lungs were under attack.

"How's the heart?" Barnard asked Coert Venter that Saturday morning.

"Fine, nothing untoward there. But he's not his usual chirpy self."

"Let's call in the team for a ten o'clock meeting," Barnard stated.

He went in to see his patient, knowing he was in some kind of trouble. Washkansky was lying on a partially-raised bed, reading glasses perched on his forehead. Next to him was a crime paperback by James Munro called *Die Rich, Die Happy*. He had dark rings under his eyes. This picture made the surgeon sad.

"Hello, Louis, how are you?"

"Awful, Doc."

His voice was hoarse and he was breathing irregularly. The indicators were not good: temperature climbing to 101.6, pulse up to 100, respiration increased from 20 to 24.

Louis complained to Barnard that he had pains in his left chest and shoulder. He reported that he was worn out.

Barnard was alarmed but tried to hide his true feelings.

He placed his stethoscope on the patient's left chest. The sounds were high-pitched, as of air being forced through a narrow tube, sure signs of tubular breathing.

"Sounds like you've caught a cold, Louis."

When he said this, Barnard couldn't look Washkansky in the eyes. Both men knew things were more serious than that. The surgeon tried to inject humour into the situation.

"Okay, Louis, no more television shows for you and no more flirting with the nurses."

Washkansky just nodded, a look of pleading in his eyes, as if he were searching for a clear statement of the truth about his condition. Barnard did not want the fighting spirit of his patient to fade and die. He didn't want the man who had been an avid sportsman for most of his life to give up and lose the zest for life for which he was known.

Back in the doctors' office, Barnard looked more closely at the latest x-ray of Washy's lungs. It was a bad picture: the tiny shadow, first identified by Dr Bosman, had magnified at least a hundred times. In addition, it was spreading from the left to the right lung. The invasion of his lungs was very rapid.

But what was causing it? It was probable he was getting pneumonia. Or a blood clot could have obstructed blood flow, leading to decay of the lung tissue. Until the cause had been confirmed, treatment could not be prescribed. But the situation was urgent, the threat growing with every passing minute. Just waiting would be dangerous. There was an unknown enemy inside Washkansky's body and unless the team could identify it and then fight it, the patient's life would soon be in the balance again.

The ten o' clock meeting in the doctors' office rapidly turned ominous in tone. Dr Forder, a finely boned, balding man with impeccable manners and a precise way of speaking, reminded the team that he'd earlier found traces of the potent bacterium Klebsiella in the patient's mouth, nostrils and rectum.

"Perhaps the patient has pneumococcal pneumonia," suggested Dr Thatcher.

"Perhaps," said Barnard, worrying that if they treated Washkansky only for pneumonia and there turned out to be a problem with blood clotting, they could lose their patient.

Professor Schrire arrived later and was convinced the problem was, indeed, pneumonia.

"How do you know for sure?" Barnard questioned.

"He looks pneumonic and his sputum is rusty," contended Schrire. "He has all the indications."

"What if it's a pulmonary infarct?"

"This is pneumonia and I believe Pencillin will wipe it out."

"Perhaps you're right."

"Trust me, I am right," Schrire claimed.

Bacteriologist Dr Forder later confirmed Schrire's diagnosis.

"We can commence Penicillin treatment," he stated.

In the ward, Washkansky's coughing was wearing him out.

Initially, the Penicillin seemed to help.

"You'll soon feel better, Louis," Barnard reassured him.

The patient said nothing in response.

"Tomorrow you should be much better," the surgeon suggested.

The medical team met for a second time in the evening and confirmed the diagnosis of pneumococcal infection. After the meeting, Barnard went back to check on Washkansky. He found Sister Papendieck in the scrub room. This was a surprise, because she was taking her first two days off since the heart operation.

"Why have you come back from your break, Sister?" he asked, gently.

She did not reply, simply shaking her head. Then she went into the ward, followed by Barnard. Their patient was sleeping and breathing heavily. His pulse had fallen to 106 but his temperature was still high at 103.8.

"What made you come back, Sister?" Barnard repeated.

Again, she did not reply. She looked down at the patient and put her hand on his bedside, once again shaking her head slowly and sadly.

"Thank you, Sister Papendieck, thank you..." was all he could say to her.

16

HOME OF HUMAN COMPASSION

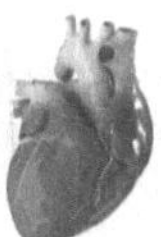

During the night, Washkansky's condition worsened and his mood sank lower. Unable to sleep, Barnard phoned Dr Coert Venter from home. Some reporters had gotten wind that something was wrong.

On Sunday, 17th December, Barnard went in early to Groote Schuur. His patient looked defeated, as if he had lost his great desire to live.

Sister Marie Papendieck was giving the patient a sponge bath. "Hello, Louis, how are you feeling?"

Washkansky shook his head.

"Come on, man, the Penicillin will start to take effect."

Breakfast was brought in for the patient but he refused to eat.

"Louis…you have to…."

"No, Doc, no. I can't do it."

Sister Papendieck stretched out a hand holding a spoonful of cereal.

"Please, Mr Washkansky, you must eat something," she pleaded.

He closed his eyes, shutting out the world.

"If you don't eat, I won't keep my dance date with you," she said.

Washkansky then picked up the spoon and began slowly eating his breakfast cereal, a gloomy look on his face.

"What's all this about a dance date?" Barnard asked, trying to inject some humour into the ward.

It was maddening to Barnard that the heart he'd transplanted into Washkansky was doing so well – no swelling, no signs of rejection – but that an unexpected lung condition was bringing the patient down. A darkening shadow was spreading right across his lungs like an omen.

At the next team meeting, it was decided to proceed with the Penicillin treatment as there had been a small reduction in the pneumococci. However, Dr Potgieter was worried that the decrease in Washkansky's white cells – from 27,390 to 24,600 – pointed to a powerful infection somewhere. In addition, for the first time, some pseudomonas, an aggressive kind of pathogen resistant to many antibiotics, had been detected. The Klebsiella bacterium had grown, too.

On Dr Forder's advice, the team added to the doses of Penicillin one gram of Cephaloridine every eight hours to combat the pseudomonas.

By evening, though, Washkansky's lungs had clogged up even more. Lesions were growing both in size and in number. The shadows on the lungs were darkening. There was no rally in the patient's condition. Soon, he was refusing to eat. A gastric tube was inserted through the nose. With his lungs under attack from a mysterious infection, it was a struggle for him just to take in air. The patient was going backwards, quickly.

It was then that his deterioration became distressing to witness. First, the fungal infection of his scrotum intensified, requiring staff to paint the affected area with gentian violet every four hours. Then he developed diarrhoea. On top of this, pain was spreading to his arms and legs.

The patient, a man of dignity, was losing his battle against sickness. Here was a man who was as brave as they come, with an intense love of life, laid low on his hospital bed. Heartbroken, Barnard worried that his spirit would soon be completely crushed.

Shortly after midnight, the surgeon went to see him again in order to provide encouragement. Washkansky was awake but looked sad and lost with all the intravenous lines and gastric tube wiring him once again to the bed and to the machinery of life support.

"Hello, Louis, how's my good man?" Barnard asked.

"I'll never get home for Christmas," the patient answered.

"There's a chance, still a chance."

"I just can't see it anymore."

"I won't give up," Barnard insisted.

"They haven't got either of us yet, have they, Doc?"

"No way," Barnard said, turning away to hide his teary eyes.

"Thank you, Louis," he said, as he turned around quickly and left the ward.

On the 15th day, there was no improvement and things were getting desperate. Bravely, Washkansky gave Barnard a weak thumbs-up sign when he greeted him that morning, showing he was still clinging on to the thread of life. But as the lung infection continued its relentless advance, he was left literally gasping for air.

Through his stethoscope, Barnard could hear the battle for life going on inside the man's chest. The patient's breath crackled, rattled and clicked. The majority of the millions of elastic air sacs, or alveoli, of Washkansky's lungs were so clogged up with fluid that air was being forced out through the popping open of small airways in irregular bursts of strangulated breath. His lungs were now in a critical condition. In response, the donor heart was pumping faster to rally to the patient's support, the pulse racing up to 110.

Despite the heart's brave efforts, however, the warm, life-giving blood was not reaching Louis's whole body. His feet and hands were turning cold. Circulation was weakening as a result of the collapsing lungs, which were sealing up with liquid.

Soon, he would suffocate.

Barnard felt pressure bearing down on him but kept his brave face on. Not only was his prize patient dying, but he was scheduled to perform another operation that day. On top of that, the US television channel CBS had informed him that they had set a date for him to appear on their prime time Face the Nation programme in the United States. Everything was threatening to get too much for him. His body was stressed, his mind stretched to the limit. He had to find a cure for Washkansky, he would not let him go!

Dr Bosman, completing night duty, came into the doctors' office, looking haggard, solemn and ashen-faced.

"We're fighting something very big here, Professor," he proclaimed.

Dr M.C. Botha, in charge of tissue matching, arrived. Taking one look at the faces of Barnard and Bosman, there was no need to ask how the world's most famous patient was faring.

"What's next?" the pathologist asked.

"I don't know," Barnard responded curtly. "Let's review where we are."

The team concluded that the treatment would have knocked out any bacterial infection, ruling out a bacterial pneumonia. They also concluded that if Washkansky's condition was caused by a viral infection, he would be beyond recovery by now.

"What about immunological pneumonia?" Barnard asked. "There are studies describing it as a side effect of the rejection process following kidney transplants. The lungs develop a condition as if they had been transplanted, not the kidneys."

Although the concept of a "ghost" transplant of this nature sounded strange to the ears of most of the scientists in the office, the hypothesis did fit with a range of facts. Dr Werbeloff confirmed that the radiological picture was not conclusive about the cause of the decline in the lungs and that this unknown immunological complication could be the culprit. Dr Forder added that he'd found no pathogenic bacteria.

"I believe Chris is correct here," stated M.C. Botha. "This is a case of a 'transplanted' lung."

The team could not get consensus because some still believed this was a case of infection, not a rejection. So Barnard went away to read up again on Hume's study of the transplanted lung to get further clarity on Washkansky's baffling condition. Refreshing himself with the details of the case study, the heart surgeon became more convinced his latest theory was correct.

He went in to see his patient. Sister Georgie Hall was changing the bed linen once again. Barnard was moved to see how much care and love was being lavished on Washkansky – and the extent of patience and perseverance shown by the nursing staff. He believed without a shadow of doubt he had the best, most caring, medical team in the whole world.

Here was the very home of human compassion.

The signs of circulatory failure were more pronounced, with blotches appearing on Washkansky's legs and arms. As a result of circulatory malfunction, his feet and hands were getting even colder.

"Louis," said Barnard, "there's still another chance left. We're starting some new treatment soon."

After that, he went back to the doctors' office and checked that Forder and Venter had not seen any fresh signs of bacteria. They had not.

"Okay, let's begin with treatment for rejection," Barnard instructed.

He prescribed strong immunosuppression drugs: 100 mgs of Hydrocortisone, 200 mgs of Actinomycin, coupled with an increase of Imuran to 250 mgs and Prednisone to 200 mgs.

Then Bosman, who'd refused to go home after his duty was over, came to Barnard to inform him it would be necessary to put Washkansky back into the oxygen tent. The capacity of the patient's blood for carrying oxygen was failing.

"That poor chap," Bossie lamented. "I remember how happy he was when we took the tent away…He felt he was rejoining the world."

"Don't be so down, man," Barnard snapped. "I want all of us to keep on believing, okay, believing that what we're doing is right."

Bosman, himself exhausted, merely nodded.

The 16th day saw a fearful deterioration in Washkansky's condition. First, he woke up that morning in a mentally confused state, making incoherent utterances. Dr Venter immediately diagnosed hypoglycaemia and gave him glucose through the nasal tube to correct the shortage of sugar in the blood.

Then it was discovered that the patient was losing white blood cells at a rate that was out of control. The count for white cells had fallen drastically from 22,200 to 5,640. Since these cells fight bacteria and destroy dead cells, this loss meant he would be increasingly powerless against his infection.

Barnard convened a crisis meeting of his team.

"This drop has occurred right after the change in therapy," reasoned Dr Potgieter, "and my hunch is that it is the Actinomycin that might be causing the problem."

It was agreed that the team would cut out the Actinomycin, as well as the Imuran. At the same time, they decided to double the dose of the anti-rejection drug, Prednisone. M.C. Botha was also asked to prepare a transfusion of white cells for the patient. The first transfusion happened early that afternoon and while it did increase the white cell count, it fell straight back again to its dangerously low level. The same thing happened with the second transfusion that evening.

Despite all the efforts, Washkansky's lungs continued to close in on him, shutting out their vital oxygen intake in a gradual suffocation. He began to turn blue. It was decided he had to be returned to artificial respiration. This meant he would no longer be able to talk. Gradually, it seemed, the house of his body was being shut down, room by room.

Barnard went into the ward to tell his patient they needed to hook him up to the respirator.

"No," he pleaded, "please, no, Doc."

"Yes, Louis. I'm sorry but it's for the best."

Washkansky shook his head and grabbed onto the sides of the oxygen tent to try to prevent them from connecting him up. He was trying to hold on to the last vestiges of control over his life. He needed his dignity, his destiny. He wanted to fend off death.

"Louis, we have to fight your lung trouble."

Washkansky looked up sorrowfully at Barnard through the plastic cover of the tent, saying nothing, still resistant.

"Louis, please keep believing in me. I believe in you. You know that, don't you?"

Dr Ozinsky came in to the ward to insert the tube through the nose and attach it to the Bird respirator. Louis closed his eyes and rolled over, defeated.

When Barnard returned to the doctors' office, he received a call from a distressed Mrs Washkansky.

"Professor, the newspaper people say Louis is dying."

"They're lying to you," Barnard retorted angrily. "Louis isn't dying, he's a fighter, remember?"

"That's who he is."

"I've got your husband on new treatment to control the lung problem."

"Oh, thank God. God bless you, Professor."

But the change to her husband's treatment could not halt the patient's decline. There was no Christmas cheer in the corridors of C-2. On the contrary, Dr Forder called Barnard at the medical school just after noon the next day, the 17th day.

"I've grown Klebsiella and pseudomonas from yesterday's sputum samples," he declared.

"I'm coming over," Barnard replied, disconsolate.

Later, in the doctors' office, Forder handed him the latest bacterial report. It made for bleak reading: "...from the sputum specimen of 19th December, heavy growths of Klebsiella and pseudomonas have been obtained. This indicates the patient is suffering from extensive bilateral pneumonia due to these organisms..."

"How could we have missed this?" Barnard asked, aghast.

"We didn't miss it," Forder replied. "It was in the oral cavity and then worked its way into the lungs."

Barnard realised at that point that the penicillin had wiped out one aggressive organism only to leave Washkansky exposed to another kind of infection. By the time the virulent Klebsiella and pseudomonas organisms had reappeared in the lungs, they had already invaded large areas of these vital organs. It had been a silent – and potentially deadly - assault. Meanwhile, the margin for recovery had by now shrunk to hours – perhaps even to minutes.

It was clear there was no time to waste. The medical team were entering the last battlefield.

Forder, Bosman and Barnard agreed that Washkansky would need a multi-pronged treatment to combat the millions of invading germs within his lungs – one gram of Carbenicillin per hour, administered through intravenous drip, plus 80 mgs of Gentamycin and two grams of Cephaloridine at intervals of eight hours each.

Scrubbing rapidly, they entered Washkansky's ward, which was now, they knew, a last chance saloon. The patient was asleep. Bosman linked up the drip for the Cephaloridine intake. Then they moved him so they could inject into his thigh the remaining antibiotics. Barnard felt the need to speak to his patient. He took his left foot and shook it gently.

"Louis! It's me, Chris Barnard, wake up."

Washkansky began to awake, wiping his eyes. His mouth opened and closed – but he could not make a sound.

"Don't worry, Louis, we've isolated the trouble in your lungs so we can treat it."

Once again, the patient tried to speak but couldn't.

"Listen, Louis, it's a question of time. You must hold on, do you hear me?"

It pained the heart surgeon to see his beloved patient so helpless.

"It's okay, Louis, I can understand you. We're here for you."

Before Washkansky's life disappeared, leaking out of him in stifled breaths, there was still some hope, however small, to find a way back. Could they heal his lungs in time? Would the remaining air pockets be able to keep him sufficiently oxygenated to stay alive? With every effort of will, and harnessing all their combined knowledge, the team were helping him to fight back. There was a tide of destruction inside him brought in by an army of microscopic germs intent on drowning out vital air sacs carrying the oxygen of life into his bloodstream.

It was now about turning back the tide of Klebsiella and pseudomonas, freeing up the lungs to pump clean air into his blood stream.

And Barnard believed the spirit of Louis, his character as a fighter, had to be part of their new counter-offensive.

"Hold on, Louis," he urged.

But there was someone else who could do a better job of encouraging Washkansky – his wife. So the medical team called her in. When she arrived, it was clear from her face that she'd been crying, her countenance seemed bruised with sadness and worry.

"It's important your husband keeps struggling, soldiering on," Barnard urged.

"Tell me what I can do, Professor. I'll do anything I can," she said.

"He has a fighting chance, a small one, but a real chance. He must know that."

Mrs Washkansky nodded tearfully.

"Keep him interested in being alive," Barnard said.

She scrubbed up and donned the gown, mask, boots and gloves and then went straight to her husband's bedside, the man who had given her a good married life, a happy, stable, fun-filled life of over twenty years together. She was distressed to see all the tubes, intravenous leads and electrode lines fixed to him. It seemed like progress had ended and they were going in reverse now.

"Louis, I'm here," she said.

He opened his eyes and nodded slowly, looking drowsy and confused.

"Please say something to me, Louis."

"He can't speak because the tube in his nose comes down his windpipe," Sister Hall explained.

After that, Ann moved closed to the bedside and bent down to talk to him, resting her hand on his pillow.

"Professor Barnard says you can make it if you don't give up, Louis. Keep fighting. Please do it for me."

At first, her husband closed his eyes but then he opened them again and moved an arm towards her. Then she took hold of his hand as if she'd been given a precious gift.

"Thank you, Louis," she said.

Then she saw he was smiling and it gladdened her to see this tiny sign of hope, of some happiness still left in his heart.

"It'll be like old times again," she told him. "You'll say, 'Let's go to Durban', and we'll get into the car and just drive and drive until we get there, just the two of us, Louis."

The medical personnel then left the couple alone, sensing it was a time for them to be alone, together.

17

OXYGENATION

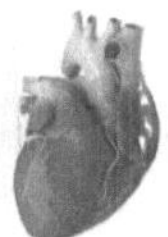

Barnard kept believing. He and his team tried everything in their power to save Louis. But some things were just beyond them. For example, the patient's white cell count decreased even more to the dangerous level of 2,790. Before the surgeon's eyes, the patient was becoming increasingly helpless against infection.

Then the flooded lungs started sending blood back into the arteries without any oxygen. The effect was dramatic: his skin began to turn a darker blue. Fortunately, at that moment, Dr Ozinsky happened to come in, cheering everyone up with his proficiency, mild manner and gentle smile.

Noting the decline in oxygenation, he decided to take Washkansky off the Bird respirator. This machine had a limit of delivering up to 40 percent oxygen. He switched the patient to a manual Boyle's anaesthetic machine. That way, Ozinsky could ventilate the lungs himself by pumping the bag as hard as he wanted, delivering up to 100 percent oxygen.

The effect of his intervention was to restore hope in the ward as the patient started to receive the right amount of oxygen. Ozzie pumped the bag at a rate of 23 times per minute. As he watched Ozinsky work the hand pump, sending pure oxygen into the depleted body of the patient, Barnard was filled with thankfulness as well as personal admiration for him. So often, during, and after, the heart operation, he'd provided moral support at critical moments.

Infused with the increased supply of oxygen, Washkansky briefly revived.

On and on, Ozinsky pumped, increasing the volume of oxygen periodically from 70 percent to 80, 90 and then 100 percent. By then, he'd reached the limit of the machine. It had become the team's last line of defence.

Midnight had descended on the ward. It had become a battleground.

"He's improving, thank goodness," Ozzie stated.

"You feel better, Louis?" he asked. "What's all this I hear about you and Sister Papendieck? I hope you're going to invite me to the party as well."

He was supplying oxygen and optimism in equal measure.

But slowly, despite his best efforts, the oxygen levels of the patient began to fall back again. The PO2 level went down to 60, then 50, then 40, falling as if over an invisible cliff. With his blood losing its oxygen content, Washkansky became blue once more.

But Ozzie didn't give up. Instead, he increased the respiration, pumping even harder, even as, inside the patient, the relentless pseudomonas aeruginosa invasion of the lungs continued unabated.

On the heart monitor, the donor heart still beat in perfect rhythm, witness to the grim deterioration of the lungs of the man it had tried to save. Beep…beep….beep. It was beating in good faith, dutiful to the end.

Barnard gazed at the regular lines of the monitor tracing the heart's strong performance, as its muscles pumped out the increasingly impure blood that would eventually kill its host.

Then he looked at the patient and found his eyes looking back into his.

"We've got to do something more," Barnard said in an uncharacteristically pleading voice. "We need time; all we need is more sweet time."

Ozzie looked up from his Boyle's pump with a quizzical expression on his face.

"How will we do that?" he asked the heart surgeon.

"We can put him back on the oxygenator," a desperate Barnard suggested.

"What good will it do, Chris?"

"It will buy us time to fight the infection. It will clean his blood."

"How much time will it give us?" Ozzie whispered. "Twelve hours, maybe twenty-four. But we've never had a man on the bypass for longer than five hours."

"I know, Ozzie, I know, but this is…different. This is Louis Washkansky. He's a fighter, remember? Who knows, maybe five hours might even be enough."

"Where will you do this, Chris?" Ozzie asked, sceptical.

"In the theatre."

"But will it really work, Prof?" Venter asked.

"I don't know for sure," Barnard answered. "Can't you guys just feel this? We can't let him die."

Feeling unsupported, he left the ward and decided to phone Val Schrire, seeking his authority to perform the task of putting Washkansky back on the heart-lung machine in the operating theatre. Even though it was 3 a.m., he didn't flinch from calling his boss at home. After a minute or two of ringing, Schrire's wife answered the phone, sounding sleepy.

"Ruth, I need to speak to Val, please?"

"He's sleeping."

"I must speak to him. It's urgent."

After a few moments, Schrire came on the line, sounding subdued.

"What is it, Chris?"

"We can't ventilate Washkansky any further. I'm considering putting him back on the oxygenator."

"On the what? Putting him back on by-pass?"

"Ja, it'll give us more time…"

"More time for what?"

"We can still beat his infection. As soon as he gets oxygen, he improves. It's a question of time."

"Chris, you don't have any time. It's all over. It was up yesterday already."

"Good God, how can you say that?"

"Listen, Chris, Mr Washkansky is dying. Clinically, he's lost. Everyone knows it except you."

Schrire's words cut through Barnard's heart like a surgeon's knife making an incision into his flesh.

"Please, Val, we've got to do something."

"To put him back on the heart-lung machine would be madness. It would merely prolong the agony – including ours, including yours, including his, including his wife's…"

Barnard was finding the conversation with his superior very difficult. He couldn't stomach this news. His mind was filled with torment. In the silence, as he tried to digest this definitive message from his superior, he wondered if he was as worried about himself – his own reputation, his own name – as much as he yearned for his patient's well-being. This thought caused him to doubt, bringing uncertainty back into play, making Schrire's words carry more authority, more weight, than his.

"Chris, are there?"

"Ja. So…you think there's no hope?"

"None. I'm sorry. There's no chance now."

"Alright, Professor. Goodbye."

Barnard hung up, a sense of hollowness falling over him. Defeat: that was what had never come easy to him. Failure had always been his biggest fear. Schrire's words had been clinically true but had sounded almost inhuman to his ears. Yet, the team's most experienced cardiologist, the man who'd founded the world-class cardiology unit at Groote Schuur, was right. Perhaps no one else in the hospital could have told

Chris Barnard to give up. But there the verdict had been given in the court of medical wisdom. The struggle was over.

Despondent and distracted, Barnard returned to the ward, pacing around aimlessly like a listless lion weary of its captivity.

"Coert," he said. "You'd better call the patient's family and tell them the news."

The first to respond to Dr Venter's call was Ann Washkansky. On her way to Groote Schuur, the patient's wife was still praying for a miracle. She still had faith, even then, that Barnard would produce something wonderful, just like the transplant itself. But this last hope was soon taken from her.

When she arrived well after 3 a.m., she saw the heart surgeon leaving her husband's ward. His hair was dishevelled and he threw his arms up.

"I don't know what to do anymore!" he cried out. "We've done everything, absolutely everything."

This reaction alarmed the patient's wife. She'd never seen the professor in such a nervous state. She began to tremble, fearing for the worst. I've had such a wonderful life with Louis, don't let him die, please God.

"It's a perfect heart, a perfect little heart," lamented Barnard, gesticulating in the corridor to his audience of two, namely Ann and himself.

"And Louis?" Ann asked.

"Louis? Your husband was brave from start to finish. I'm just so ashamed we couldn't save him."

There was so much sorrow and torment on the surgeon's face, she began to feel sorry for him. But the whole encounter had frightened her.

"Is he dead?" she asked.

"No, not that," he mumbled, shuffling away down the corridor in a distracted state of mind.

Ann went straight into the scrub room but she was so upset she forgot to put the gloves and mask on. When she entered the ward, Dr Venter was in the corner and Sister Papendieck was at the bedside like a guardian angel. Washkansky was barely alive, blue, cold, his eyes glazed.

"Louis, it's me, Ann. Louis, I've come to be with you."

No response. Ann decided to talk to her husband, hoping he could hear even if he could no longer speak.

"Tell me, Louis, what I can do for you. I'm here to help."

Washkansky lay motionless on his death bed. She moved closer in line with his eyes so he could see her better. But there was no flicker of love, or life, in his eyes. Then she realised her hands were bare and she could touch him properly, skin on skin, for the first time since his momentous operation over a fortnight ago. It was too late to worry about germs so she touched his face and his hands and his arms, her love passing into his cool, blue body, caressing him softly. He looked so lonely, so isolated in his advanced state of decline.

"We've got a wonderful marriage, Louis, you and I," she told him. "So many memories, so many laughs…You've been so good to me, darling man."

Still, there was no response. The only movement was from Sister Papendieck pumping the anaesthetic machine to keep him alive.

"I'm staying with you, Louis. I'm not going away now."

Ann looked to the side and saw the Sister's face and mask were wet with tears.

"Let me help, Sister, let me pump for him a little bit."

Soon, she was joined in the ward by her brother and other members of the Washkansky family. In the solemn quiet and sterility of the hospital room, they paid their last respects. However, when the patient's stomach began to swell, the medical team told the visitors they needed to leave.

"I can help," Ann protested, "I can stay and help Sister Papendieck."

"No," her brother told her, "you need to help your son Michael, he's locked himself in the car outside."

"But what if Louis calls for me?" she answered, fretting.

"Michael needs you much more now than Louis," her brother replied, and his words seemed to carry wisdom, showing Ann and the family the right thing to do at that moment.

One by one, they greeted the silent, unresponsive man they loved. Then they filed out of the room.

Still in an abstracted state of mind, Barnard watched them leave the building from the window of the ward. He saw Washkansky's red Zephyr below in the parking lot next to his own car, under a large palm tree. Inside, their young son Michael was weeping. Barnard thought of his own father, Adam, the small town minister of religion and missionary to the Coloured people of Beaufort West, and how strong he'd always been for all his sons despite his social and financial struggles. He could only wonder at the grief flooding Michael's young mind as his father's life began to finally fade away into the dark emptiness of death.

He saw Ann knock on the window of their Zephyr.

"Michael, we have to talk, please open the door," she said.

But there really wasn't much to talk about when he unlocked the doors, because the boy knew that what he needed to help him most would not be words of cold comfort but rather the actual memories of his father, of the good times they'd had together, of how strong he'd seemed to his son whenever he'd held him or picked him up, of how the love and the strength of his father had mysteriously flowed into him then...The motor of the car started up and broke the silence at the end of night. Then they left, going down the hill into the dark suburbs flickering with the last of the night lights. A few moments later, some of the streetlights and house lights began to blink off in the distance out across the Cape Flats as a new day brushed the horizons with a glowing grey, soft as muted watercolours.

18

"IF MR DARVALL SAID 'YES', HOW CAN I SAY 'NO'?"

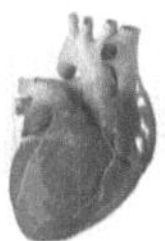

Ozzie, Sister Papendieck and Coert Venter took turns to pump the machine to keep Washkansky alive. No one had told them to stop doing what they did best – caring, giving, helping, loving.

Then Washkansky's circulation slowed even more. The team administered calcium intravenously but it provided no relief. The patient's blood continued to cool and to deteriorate in quality, low in oxygen and nutrients, concentrated with urea and waste, turning dark. As a result, Louis's skin seemed even darker, cold and increasingly lifeless with a sickly bluish tinge. His diseased lungs were draining life out of his body, the shadow of death was spreading further across him with each passing minute, despite the healthy donor heart which had given him a rebirth, followed by eighteen extra days of life.

The end came when the heart, deprived of its critical partnership with the lungs, could no longer cope with the flood of deoxygenated blood. Around 6.30 a.m. the heart that had once beat inside Denise Darvall began to malfunction in its new host body. The line on the heart monitor became more erratic, the beeps of the machine getting louder and more strident. Cardiac arrhythmia set in. Disorder was increasing, beyond the power to control. As the new summer day broke, death approached.

"Professor, the transplanted heart is taking strain, it's in fibrillation now," Coert announced.

The line of the heart on the machine was erratic. Then its flow ceased, abruptly flatlining across the screen. His patient, their patient, the whole world's patient, had breathed his last.

Sister Papendieck cried.

"I want to thank you all," Barnard said, his voice trembling, his eyes fixed on the monitor to reinforce the evidence he didn't want to believe: that his patient had died. "You've been wonderful."

He went out into the porch to be alone, sadness clouding his eyes, sorrow clutching at his throat. He wanted to get away, to go somewhere quiet, but he bumped into Dr Bosman on his way out.

"We need to arrange a post-mortem," Bosman stated.

"Yes, of course," Barnard replied, numbly.

"I'll call Professor Thomson and Dr Forder immediately."

"Alright, that would be good."

With that duty taken care of, Barnard wandered outside to get some fresh air. He didn't want to get into his car so he just started walking, trying to absorb the shock of the loss of Washkansky, all the more cruel and ironic because he'd died of lung disease, not any failure of his transplanted heart.

Walking down the hill towards the main road of Observatory, he started to collect his thoughts. The most famous patient in the world had died, and, with him, the hope he'd brought to millions. Death had stolen a good man, a life-loving man, a wife-loving man, a people-loving man.

Coincidentally, Barnard passed the old cemetery on Main Road at this time, which was on a plot adjacent to the hospital. Its grey gravestones seemed gloomy among the soft, ghostly grass. He turned into a lane which led past the animal laboratory where he, Marius and Naki had carried out transplantation experiments on stray dogs and baboons. Just behind the lab, was the post-mortem theatre where Washkansky's cadaver would shortly be examined. Further down the lane, Barnard came to his medical offices, arriving there just after 7.30 a.m. This is where the international media siege had largely played out during the aftermath of the operation. Now, its corridors and offices were empty and still.

In his secretary's office, next to the phone which hadn't stopped ringing in the heady days after the transplant, was a copy of the latest edition of Time Magazine. It was dated December 15, 1967, priced at fifty cents. On the front cover was a colour portrait of Barnard by American artist Robert Vickrey, who'd been drawing for the magazine for a decade, against a background of a bright red heart and its vessels and arteries cascading behind the surgeon's head. The caption, diagonally placed across the top left corner of the front cover read simply: The Transplanted Heart.

Barnard noticed that the ring of a coffee cup, which had stood on the news magazine, stained the picture, as if to bring him back down to earth from the giddy heights of being an international name. He looked critically at himself and felt alienated from the whole coverage of this great episode in his life, now ended in the anti-climax of apparent failure.

Idly, he flicked through the correspondence in his in-tray, telegrams, letters and invitations from around the world to appear at medical conferences, universities and civic groups. Little did they all know when they penned the invitations how grim Washkansky's passing had been, his life swallowed up by the microscopic pathogens which had swarmed into his lungs, engulfing its air sacs, resistant to the best treatment the hospital had to offer.

But then Barnard's eye was caught by the letter from CBS confirming that the US broadcaster had finalised all the arrangements for a panel discussion on a Christmas Eve special edition of Face the Nation, along with Dr Michael De Bakey and Dr Adrian Kantrowitz. He looked on his desk calendar – the broadcast was only four days away. What was he to do? Wouldn't it appear cowardly and defeatist if he turned down the chance to appear on the high-profile news show, bringing shame to his team, his hospital and his nation?

The urgency of this question woke him up from the slumber of his intense sadness, inspiring a new train of thought in his mind. Yes, he was deflated, it was true. But was he really defeated? Hang on, Boetie, just look at all this interest from the four corners of the world? And hadn't a window in heaven opened up eighteen days ago when hope was first given to terminally ill heart patients at Groote Schuur's cardiac unit?

At once, Barnard knew he had no choice but to accept the invitation from CBS. He'd make plans immediately to return to the United States. It was in America a decade ago, while a post-graduate medical student, that his dream of pioneering heart transplant surgery in his homeland had been born. Not only that, he would return to this country not as a loser but as a winner, as a country boy whose improbable dream of changing the medical world forever had come true in Ward C2 of Groote Schuur, Cape Town's fortress of medicine.

The surgeon's thoughts were interrupted by a knock at the door. It was a colleague who'd been a rival registrar at the start of their careers, Dr Jacques Roux.

"I heard it on the radio, Chris, I'm so damn sorry."

So the world knew already, Barnard thought to himself. Louis Washkansky was dead.

"I crash-landed," Barnard said.

"No, you opened up a new way," Roux responded.

"I gave the man too many anti-rejection drugs. His resistance suffered – he couldn't fight the infection. We tried to…"

Barnard felt relief as he shared this confession, adding to the more positive frame of mind he'd started to build inside himself just before Roux arrived.

"I know, Chris. But you were feeling your way in the dark. That's how it works in medicine. You stole light from the darkness."

"I'm not yet sure if I can ever do it again, Jacques."

"You have no choice, you can't give up now. You must do another heart transplant."

Before Barnard could reply, the phone rang. It was Dr Bosman, informing him that the post-mortem on Washkansky was about to commence.

"Bossie, you know, Jewish law doesn't allow mutilation of the dead body."

"I know, I've already spoken to Ann Washkansky," Bosman answered. "We've got her permission."

"Thank you, that's good. What did she say, then?"

"She said, 'If Mr Darvall said 'yes', how can I say 'no'?'"

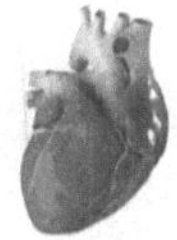

Did the 1967 medical breakthrough fulfill a 2,600 year old prophecy?

*An analysis of history's first human heart transplant
in the light of Ezekiel 11:19*

"All mankind stands at this moment at the graveside of Louis Washkansky – may his grave be for a blessing."

PROFESSOR I. ABRAHAMS, CHIEF RABBI
OF THE CAPE, AT THE FUNERAL OF LOUIS
WASHKANSKY, PINELANDS, 22 DECEMBER
1967

It seems that the story of the first human heart transplant, which took place in the early hours of 3rd December 1967 at

Groote Schuur Hospital in Cape Town, South Africa, may be about to yield yet another twist, 50 years on.

The priest Ezekiel, one of three major Old Testament prophets (the other two being Isaiah and Jeremiah), recorded some 2,600 years ago what can only be described as a startling piece of foreknowledge, namely, that transplants of human organs would become part of medicine in the future:

I will remove from them their heart of stone and give them a heart of flesh.

EZEKIEL 11:19

The context of this ancient scripture is the promised return of the people of Israel from their exile in Babylon which began in 597 B.C. The passage in which it occurs is highly literary and prophetical, with a positive tone established through a series of promises for the future. Although Ezekiel 11:19 anticipates a spiritual rebirth, it does draw an analogy between this process of inner renewal and an organ transplant. It paints a picture of the actual removal of a defective heart and its replacement with a living, or healthy, heart, which points to the medical purpose of a heart transplant.

The new translation of the Afrikaans Bible brings out the vividness of Ezekiel's figure of speech:

Ek sal die kliphart uit hulle liggam verwyder en hulle 'n hart van vleis gee.

Underlying such a comparison between a spiritual and physical transplant is the startling insight of an ancient prophecy that it will become possible in the future of medicine to remove inner organs from the body and replace them with ones which are in better condition.

Ezekiel, who was prophesying to his fellow exiled Jews (1), wanted, then, to illustrate the spiritual equivalent of what we call today a heart transplant. But medical knowledge itself only caught up with the underlying concept of Ezekiel 11:19 over two and a half thousand years later. That was when heart surgeon Professor Christiaan Barnard, his brother Marius and the whole heart team at Groote Schuur Hospital, placed the heart of Denise Darvall, who had just been declared brain-dead after a motor vehicle accident, into the body of a dying man called Louis Washkansky on that fateful weekend early in December of '67.

It's important to conduct some exegesis on this text to make sure the right conclusions are being drawn from it. An exegesis is defined as "a thorough, analytical study of a biblical passage done so as to arrive at a useful interpretation of the passage." (2) The idea is to determine the specific meaning of a scripture, properly contextualised and using lexical analysis of key words like "heart", "flesh", "stony" and "remove".

The Hebrew word for "remove", or take out, here is *cûwr*, originally meaning to turn off, with other meanings like pluck away, remove, be without, withdraw, etc. It can even have connotations of deterioration. In this verse, the verb indicates getting rid of something. The word "stony", which translates *eben*, from the root word in Hebrew for build, *bânâh*, suggests that the organ in question is completely lifeless, especially when compared to a heart of flesh. The word "flesh" occurs twice in the verse as shown in the King James Version:

> I will take the stony heart out of their flesh, and will give them a heart of flesh.

In both occurrences of the word, the Hebrew is *bâsâr*, derived from the verb to be fresh, to be full (cheerful), the idea being that flesh is fresh or healthy. Other applications of the meaning include the body, the person, nakedness, the self and skin. The word "flesh" in the scripture clearly refers, then, to a dimension of the physical body.

To paraphrase in a transliterated sense, this verse is talking about getting rid of something rotten or defective in the body as part of a broader spiritual analogy.

The Hebrew word for "heart" in Ezekiel 11:19 is *lêb* or *lêbâb*, referring to the body's most interior, or enclosed, organ, with a wide range of possible applications such as the centre of something, the will, the intellect, the feelings and what we might call today the soul, mind or seat of intelligence and consciousness. It should be remembered in exegesis that a "single Hebrew word rarely corresponds precisely to a single English word but may range in meaning through all or parts of several English words." (3)

The New Bible Dictionary points out that this Old Testament word "heart" (lêb) can refer to the internal organs as well, as we see when it occurs in the graphic description of the death of Absalom:

So, he [Joab] took three javelins in his hand and plunged them into Absalom's heart while Absalom was still alive in the oak tree.

In New Testament Greek, the word for heart is *kardia*, meaning the chief organ of physical life (Vine's *Expository Dictionary of New Testament Words*), which was often used figuratively to refer to "the hidden springs of the personal life". (4)

The point about this kind of figurative language, of course, is that a figure of speech typically sets up a comparison between something literal and a meaning the writer is trying to describe, as in "my love is like a red, red rose" in the Robert Burns poem or "Shall I compare thee to a summer's day?" in the opening line of the well-known Shakespearean sonnet. A comparison, according to *The New Oxford Dictionary of English*, is a "consideration or estimate of the similarities or dissimilarities between two things or people." (5)

To return to Ezekiel 11:19, the prophet is comparing a spiritual revival to the physical removal of an interior organ, even though at the time the concept of a heart transplant would have been completely inconceivable. That is why it appears we are dealing with a case of foreknowledge, that is, knowing about something before it happens or has become real. One scholar observes that Ezekiel possessed "unique powers of telepathy, clairvoyance and prognosis." (6) Another Old Testament scholar described the prophet as combining ecstatic visions of the future with a sober sense of reality. (7) We see Ezekiel's powers of foretelling the future on display in his prediction of a future restoration of the state of Israel following exile:

> This is what the Sovereign Lord says: I will take the
> Israelites out of the nations where they have gone. I
> will gather them from all around and bring them
> back into their own land. I will make them one
> nation in the land, on the mountains of Israel. There
> will be one king over all of them and they will never
> again be two nations or be divided into two
> kingdoms.
>
> EZEKIEL 37:21-22

As a professional priest and a prophet whose ministry lasted over two decades, Ezekiel remains a towering biblical figure. His vision of a heart transplant centuries before it became factual must rank as one of the greatest prognostications of human history. It is evident that the 1967 human heart transplant turned the concept behind this comparison made by Ezekiel between spiritual and physical heart transplants into a fact.

In an historic operation lasting close to six hours, Chris Barnard and his team removed the dying heart of Louis Washkansky ("stony heart") and replaced it with the healthy heart of donor Denise Darvall ("heart of flesh"). What is truly remarkable is that the '67 medical breakthrough, which perhaps fulfilled a 2,600 year-old biblical promise, saw the heart of a gentile woman placed into the body of a dying Jewish man, a symbolic event of reconciliation with important historical and religious overtones. When Louis Washkansky died 18 days after the very first human heart transplant, the woman's heart inside him was still performing beautifully. The post mortem showed that the cause of death had been respiratory failure brought about by double pneumonia following the invasion of his lungs by the dangerous klebsiella bacterium.

Time Magazine in Africa journalist Peter Hawthorne, author of the first book about the operation, *The Transplanted Heart*, wrote in 1968 that the rabbinical authorities he consulted, including Dr Immanuel Jakobovitz, Chief Rabbi of the British Commonwealth, all concluded that there had been no transgression of Jewish religious law in the transplant of an Anglican Christian woman into the body of Washkansky, a Jewish businessman. (8)

Chris and Marius Barnard had themselves grown up in a devout Christian home. Their father Adam was employed as a minister to the Coloured people in the Dutch Reformed Church in Beaufort West. At the end of his autobiography, Marius Barnard wrote: "Throughout my life I have striven to embody the ideals embraced by my father, whose passionate belief in God, compassion and the resilience of the human spirit was matched only by his boundless love for children....Unlike Frank Sinatra, who sings that he did it his way, I can, now that my end is near, say with total conviction that I did it God's way." (9) While not as religious as his parents or his younger brother, what is not very well-known about Chris Barnard is that he, too, was a man of faith who prayed before major operations, including while he was showering before the historic heart operation. In his autobiography *One Life* he testified that he derived strength from prayer. "I could never sustain my life, nor nourish the memory of my father," he wrote, "if I did not believe in God." (10)

So, this act of symbolic reconciliation between two faiths, and between the female and male genders, in the 1967 heart operation, led by men of prayer, carried no religious or theological offence. It does strike me as compelling that this kind of message is part of the meaning of an operation that turned the medical promise underlying an ancient prophecy into a fact of modern science.

Notes

1) Wolff, Hans Walter. *The Old Testament: A Guide to its Writings*. London: SPCK (1974). 96-7.

"Ezekiel made his appearance in 593 B.C. in Babylon among the exiles who belonged to the first group that had been deported in 597. His writings give us the most precise indications of how the proclamation of God's judgment on Jerusalem was transformed into the expectation of salvation, once the city had been destroyed."

2) Stuart, Douglas. *Old Testament Exegesis: A primer for students and pastors*. Philadelphia: The Westminster Press (1980). 15.
3) Stuart, Douglas. *Old Testament Exegesis: A primer for students and pastors*. Philadelphia: The Westminster Press (1980). 25.
4) Vine's Expository Dictionary of New Testament Words. Oliphants Ltd (1952).
5) The New Oxford Dictionary of English. Oxford: Oxford University Press (1998). 373.
6) ed. Guthrie, D, Motyer, JA, Stibbs, AM and Wiseman, DJ. *New Bible Commentary* (Third Edition). Leicester: Inter- Varsity Press (1970). 666.
7) Fohrer, G. *Introduction to the Old Testament*. London: SPCK (1986). 415.
8) Hawthorne, P. *The Transplanted Heart*. Johannesburg: Hugh Keartland Publishers (1968). 146.
9) Barnard, M & Norval, S. *Defining Moments*. Cape Town: Zebra Press (2011). 407.
10) Barnard, CN & Pepper, CB. *One Life*. Cape Town: Howard Timmins (1969). 155.

Other References

Strong's Exhaustive Concordance of the Bible. Nashville: Abingdon Press (1986)

The New International Version and the King James Version

AFTERWORD

Reflecting on the Life and Times of Hamilton Naki: animal laboratory surgeon extraordinaire

By Anwar Suleman Mall, Acting Deputy Vice Chancellor and Professor, Division of General Surgery, UCT, Grant Willis, Director of Student Housing, UCT, and Michael Lee, author of *Heartbeat*

It's a story which could only have happened in South Africa. Hamilton Naki (1926-2005) was a son of the Eastern Cape who rose from menial work to become a highly skilled, largely self- taught laboratory experimental surgeon, able to perform complex operations on animals in the JS Marais Animal Laboratory at UCT's medical school, all without high-school education or formal medical qualifications (1,2).

In the groundbreaking years of the early 1960s, he worked as an assistant with the Barnard brothers in this laboratory where the skills needed to carry out subsequent human heart transplants were honed to near-perfection. As such, Naki forms a unique part

of the historical kaleidoscope of innovation in transplantation at Groote Schuur Hospital which, in 1967, truly lit up the medical world.

It should be noted at the outset, however, that, according to all the records, including the autobiographical accounts of this historic operation by both Chris and Marius Barnard (4,5), that he played *no part whatsoever* in the world's first human heart transplant of 1967. Nor did he participate in *any* subsequent surgery on human beings at Groote Schuur Hospital. His work was wholly confined to this important experimental laboratory of animal surgery. Indeed, given this historical fact, it's regrettable that Mr Naki's image was, in part, tarnished posthumously and unnecessarily, due to misconceptions in the media, and elsewhere in the public domain, about the precise nature of his involvement in the heart-transplant programme. The reality is that he was never directly involved in any human surgery.

Hamilton Naki should thus be best remembered in posterity as an animal laboratory surgeon *extraordinaire*.

Hamilton grew up poor in the humble Xhosa village of Centani in what was then called Transkei. After completing primary school, he set out for the metropolis of Cape Town as an economic migrant. Armed only with a Standard Six (Grade 8) education and living by his wits as a teenager far from home, he was hired by the University of Cape Town to maintain the grass of the university's lawn tennis courts (3).

It was around 1954 that he got his breakthrough when he was approached to take care of animals in the animal medical laboratory (2). It appears he began with menial tasks like cleaning cages and weighing animals. Later, he got involved in putting up drips, stitching and even anaesthetising the animals, evolving, in the process, into a fully-fledged laboratory technician.

Just being in this hotbed of scientific development at the medical school must have fired his imagination and his passion for experimental medical research. Instinctively, he sensed he was gifted enough to develop himself further in this field. Hamilton Naki had found his life's niche.

Meanwhile, Chris Barnard had returned to South Africa in 1958 from his doctoral studies at the University of Minnesota, Minneapolis, USA, along with a groundbreaking piece of medical technology, a heart-lung machine. It was later used in the first human heart transplant operation (4).

When Barnard began his pioneering work on organ transplants on dogs, Naki was the anaesthetist. In this period, Marius Barnard performed numerous surgical operations at the animal laboratory, in preparation for the human heart transplants. At the time, laboratory technician Victor Pick, a Capetonian, served as the leader of lab assistants (2, 4).

Naki continued to progress, eventually assisting with, and performing, transplants on the animals, including cardiac and liver transplants. He worked on baboons, rabbits and pigs as well as dogs. He was especially knowledgeable about liver transplants. In his autobiography, Marius Barnard, who performed about 90% of the operations on dogs, taken from the local pound, prior to 1967, writes that, in his understanding, Naki's liver transplant research after 1967 was "comparable to that of a trained surgeon" (5).

Although he never performed surgery on human patients in operating theatres, it could be fairly said that the animal laboratory work, in which Naki played a critical role, contributed to the success of Groote Schuur Hospital's world-famous human heart operations. In his autobiography, Chris Barnard mentioned that after this laboratory had carried out about 25 operations on dogs, he felt ready to accept the risk of transplanting a human

heart (4).

In addition to the subtle dexterity of his fingers, his large hands able to move with a distinct nimbleness, Naki must have possessed an extraordinarily intuitive understanding of anatomy. He learnt not from text books but from direct observation. When asked by a reporter how he managed to learn these skills without a formal education, he replied "I stole with my eyes." (1)

On top of his natural gift for grasping the intricate anatomical structure of animals, coupled with his budding surgical skills, he must have been a daring individual to undertake numerous difficult operations on so many creatures.

His status as full laboratory technician was confirmed in the mid-1980s after an administrative evaluation at UCT. Grant Willis, now the University's Director of Student Housing, had been tasked to interview an employee apparently carrying out heart transplants on animals. Rather amazed to hear this, Willis went down the University Medical School in search of this employee. There, he was ushered into an operating theatre.

"I saw lots of medical equipment in the theatre and an operating table with lights directly over it and a gentleman dressed in a white laboratory coat," Willis recalls. "This was Hamilton Naki. He waved me over to the operating table, which I approached cautiously. On the table, covered by a white sheet, was an animal I couldn't identify. The sheet covered most of the animal except for a small section that had been left open. As I peered into this section, I saw the insides of the animal and, most prominently, the creature's heart."

Fascinated, Willis drew closer to view the proceedings.

"I noticed clamps and other medical instruments around the heart as Hamilton proceeded to inform me in some detail how he carried out a heart transplant. I was astounded that this employee

was really performing heart transplants."

As a result of the administrative evaluation submitted by Willis after this memorable interview, and later ratified by management, Naki's grade was advanced from Departmental Assistant to full laboratory technician, befitting his high level of skill (Grant Willis's email communication).

The surgeon from Langa was thriving, succeeding beyond his wildest dreams. And he'd progressed by a combination of will-power, force of personality and detailed, first-hand knowledge he'd picked up over many years in the Animal Laboratory.

Naki had overcome the limits of his aborted school education, as well as the crippling restrictions of Apartheid, on his path of progress. But he didn't stop there. He then proceeded to pass on his knowledge to numerous medical trainees, deepening his legacy (2).

He didn't know it then, but as a result of his achievements and dedication to the cause of experimental research, here were the makings of another future legend of South Africa's medical profession from this distinctively innovative period.

As a man, Naki was reported to be impeccably mannered and well-dressed, with a warm-hearted demeanour. He evidently possessed a deep reservoir of humanity and humour. Despite his achievements in the medical field, he remained humble, and was known in private to be a devout person, an avid reader of the Bible, a copy of which he often had in his possession (1,2).

In 2002, Hamilton Naki received South Africa's civilian honour of the Bronze Order of Mapungubwe (medical science) (2). Then, in the following year, he was awarded an honorary Master of Medicine degree from UCT (2).

Upon retiring from Groote Schuur, he received the pension

of a Senior Laboratory Assistant, living out his final years peacefully at his home in Langa, Cape Town.

The story of Hamilton Naki is one of the most remarkable examples of personal progress from poverty this country has experienced.

Extraordinary achievements aren't measured by success alone but by how far a person has come in his, or her, life's journey, and which obstacles were overcome along the way. Naki's rise from economic migrant and school drop-out to self-taught surgeon at the Animal Laboratory of a leading academic hospital, in that particular momentous time, is a phenomenon South Africa can celebrate with pride for generations to come.

1. Mall, A.S. *Hamilton Naki, a surgical Sherpa.* SAMJ Forum July 2006, Vol.96, No.7.
2. Cotton, M, Hickman, R and Mall, A.S. *Hamilton*

Naki, his life, and his role in the first heart transplant. Royal College of Surgeons of England Bulletin. 2014; 96;1-4.

3. Hickman, R. *From tennis courts to transplants.* Arch Surg 1999; 134:451-452.

4. Barnard, C & Pepper, Curtis. 1969. *One Life.* Cape Town: Howard Timmins.

5. Barnard, M & Norval, S. 2011. *Defining Moments.* Cape Town: Zebra Press.

6. http://www.sahistory.org.za/people/hamilton-naki South African History Online

ACKNOWLEDGMENTS

Heartbeat is a fact-based account of the first human heart transplant, a stirring event in medical history which took place on 3rd December 1967 in Cape Town. This documentary novel naturally relied on sources like Peter Hawthorne's 1968 book *The Transplanted Heart* and the essay in Time Magazine in the edition which appeared in the same month as the transplant, as well as the autobiographical works of the Barnard brothers, Chris and Marius, namely *One Life* and *Defining Moments*, respectively. Equally useful was the information and memorabilia on display in such commemorative locations as the Heart of Cape Town Museum, the Chris Barnard Museum in Beaufort West and the Christiaan Barnard Memorial Hospital, including newspaper cuttings of the time.

This is a story deeply embedded in the fabric of South African history and in the psyche of the nation. Most works describing, or alluding to, the transplant and to the life of Chris Barnard have, however, focused on the sensational above the factual. The facts surrounding the operation are incredible enough, as you will soon see, without the need for any kind of embellishment. Accordingly, this novel is grounded firmly in the real medical drama of the transplant itself.

I would like to thank my wife Sannettha for her belief in this project and for her careful and caring research into the large cast of real characters you are about to meet. I am grateful to the management and staff of the Heart of Cape Town Museum at Groote Schuur Hospital for their review of the manuscript of *Heartbeat* to check its accuracy. I would like to thank Bruce Mathew, a leading Neurosurgeon at Hull & East Yorkshire Hospitals NHS Trust, United Kingdom, for his deeply insightful appraisal of the draft manuscript from both the medical and narrative points of view.

This true story is dedicated to the Barnards. Their rise from poverty to power and influence really begins long before 1967, on a summer's day near the end of the 19th century, when Adam Hendrikus Barnard walked out of the forests of Knysna to leave behind for good the grinding existence of a wood-cutter, to which he'd been born, in order to seek a new life for himself and his descendants, including the son who would one day change the world.

REVIEW

BY NEUROSURGEON, DR BRUCE MATHEW

We are all familiar with the story of the first human heart transplant. Michael Lee has brought this tale to life with fascinating insights into the lives of the key people involved. Instead of just lauding the surgeons, he has rightly venerated the heroism of nursing staff, patients, donors and their families. In hindsight, the establishment of brain death is arguably the most significant legacy left by these pioneering heart surgeons. The concept of the heart as 'just a wonderful pump' has averted much unnecessary suffering by allowing life support to be discontinued when brain death criteria have been met, indicating the futility of further active management. Transplantation surgery has been a positive consequence of this conceptual shift and 'brain death' is now a pillar of modern medical thinking.

Since this historic operation, organ donation has become common practice. To illustrate this point, in the UK alone every kidney transplant saves the NHS in the region of £1 million pounds, by avoiding the need for dialysis. We have performed brain surgery on several patients, living normal lives, after having had heart transplants. One of my colleagues enjoyed a high quality of life for many years after a heart/lung transplant. Most body parts have now been successfully transplanted. Brain

transplantation itself cannot happen as one would need a new body, given that the personhood of an individual really inheres in the brain.

The narrative also has some personal connections. Michael and I were both at Rondebosch Boys' High School in the Cape, as was Adam, son of Marius Barnard, a surgeon in the famous heart team who recently passed away. I was at UCT medical school and Groote Schuur Hospital from 1974 to 1983 so most of the people mentioned in this book were my teachers and respected senior colleagues.

Rodney Hewitson and his family have been my long-standing friends. Rodney's son John has followed in his father's footsteps and works at Red Cross Children's hospital as a respected cardio thoracic surgeon. And my mother's uncle was a minister in a similar church to Christian Barnard's father, in this case situated near George and hence the Knysna forests where the ancestors of the Barnard family had lived for generations as humble forest- dwellers and wood-cutters.

I very much hope this inspiring true story resonates with you and that you enjoy the narrative as much as I have done.

Dr Bruce Mathew
November 2014

LIST OF CHARACTERS

Main characters

Professor Christiaan Barnard, heart surgeon at Groote Schuur Hospital

Louis Washkansky, recipient of the world's first transplanted human heart

Dr Marius Barnard, cardiac surgeon and younger brother of Chris

Denise Ann Darvall, heart donor for the heart transplant

Professor Val Schrire, founder and head of Groote Schuur's cardiac unit

Dr "Bossie" Bosman, registrar at Groote Schuur cardiac unit ***Dr Coert Venter***, surgeon in Chris Barnard's heart team ***Sister Marie Papendieck***, senior nursing sister at cardiac unit ***Dr Joseph Ozinsky***, senior anaesthetist in the heart team

Dr Rodney Hewitson, heart surgeon and senior assistant to Chris Barnard

Mrs Ann Washkansky, wife to Louis Washkansky

Additional characters

Dr Peter Rose-Innis, neurosurgeon at Groote Schuur tasked to decide whether Denise Darvall had been rendered brain-dead after being knocked down by a drunken driver

Dr M.C.Botha, pathologist, immunologist and member of the heart team

Sister Peggy Jordaan, instrument sister during heart transplant

Mrs Louwtjie Barnard, wife of Chris Barnard

Deirdre Barnard, daughter of Chris and Louwtjie Barnard ***Andre 'Boetie' Barnard,*** son of Chris and Louwtjie Barnard ***Edward Darvall***, father of Denise Darvall

Myrtle Darvall, mother of Denise Darvall

Keith Darvall, brother of Denise Darvall, witness to the accident

Hamilton Naki, animal laboratory surgeon at JS Marais Animal Laboratory at UCT's medical school

Victor Pick, lab leader at JS Marais Animal Laboratory

Travelling salesman, driver of the car which killed Myrtle and Denise Darvall

Dr Louis Ehrlich, physician who examined Denise Darvall at the scene of the accident

Fred Jones Munnik and Jan Marais, drivers of Ambulance Number 16 from Pinelands depot which took the crash victims to Groote Schuur Hospital

Ann Taibal, sister-in-law of Ann Washkansky

Tevia Washkansky, brother of Louis Washkansky

Gracie Sklar, Washkansky's sister-in-law

Chavia Taibel, Washkansky's niece

Solly Sklar, Washkansky's brother-in-law and old friend

Ann, Washkansky's older sister

Michael Washkansky, son of Louis Washkansky

Dr Jacques Roux, surgeon and long-standing colleague of Chris Barnard at Groote Schuur

Dr Barry Kaplan, Washkansky's physician

Dr Bernard Pimstone, physician treating Washkansky's diabetes

Dr Francois Hitchcock, surgeon and member of heart team

Dr Terry O'Donovan, surgeon and member of the heart team

Dr Cecil Moss, second anaesthetist in B Theatre during transplant, and former Springbok rugby player and coach

Dr Gideon Potgieter, biochemist and part of Chris Barnard's team of post-operative team of experts and specialists

Dr Arderne Forder, bacteriologist and part of the post-operative team of experts and specialists

Dr Geoff Thatcher, nephrologist and part of the post-operative team of experts and specialists

Dr J.G. Burger, medical superintendent of Groote Schuur Hospital at time of heart transplant

Dr Johan de Klerk, performed kidney transplant at Karl Bremer Hospital, using Denise Darvall's donated kidney

Johan van Heerden, Dene Friedman, Nic Vermaak and Alistair Hope, pump technicians on the heart-lung machines during heart transplant

Sisters Tollie Lambrechts, Georgie Hall, Fox-Smith, Kingsley, Amelia Rautenbach and Sannie Rossouw, nursing sisters at Groote Schuur's cardiac unit

Professor Lennox Eales, head of renal unit at Groote Schuur at time of heart transplant

Professor James Thomson, head of pathology at the University of Cape Town at the time of the transplant

Professor James Kench, biochemist and part of the team of post-operative experts and specialists

Dr Simcha Banks, bacteriologist and part of the team of post- operative experts and specialists

Dr Leslie Werbeloff, radiologist and part of the team of post- operative experts and specialists

Mrs Ruth Schrire, wife of Professor Val Schrire

Professor Jannie Louw, head of department of surgery at Groote Schuur

Rabbi Israel Abrahams, Washkansky's rabbi

Gerald Ferry, major of Cape Town at the time of the transplant and old acquaintance of Washkansky's

Edith Black, recipient of Chris Barnard's successful kidney transplant of 1967

Paul John Thesen, world's longest surviving heart transplant patient, operated on 5 January 1979 at Groote Schuur (died December 2013)

Reporters and journalists from international mass media

Heart of Cape Town Museum

Groote Schuur Hospital, Main Road, Observatory, South Africa

www.heartofcapetown.co.za | info@heartofcapetown.co.za

Tel : +27 21 404 1967

The Chris Barnard Museum – Die Pastorie

Gracia Street, Beaufort West, Karoo, South Africa, 6970

Tel : +27 23 415 2308

Support the Christiaan Barnard Heart Foundation

(www.cbheartfoundation.com)

ABOUT THE AUTHOR

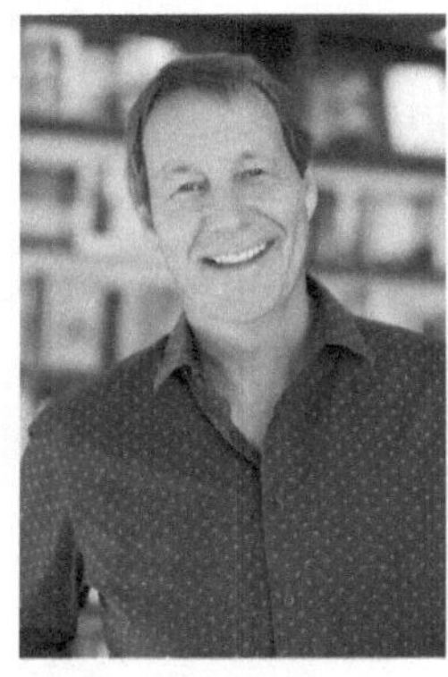

Michael enjoys reading, writing, painting, sketching, jogging and watching powerful movies, having built up a private collection of several hundred DVDs and Blu-ray films spanning the entire history of cinema to the present. He has been married to Sannettha since 1990 and the couple have two daughters, Michaela, a food and cosmetic scientist, and Melissa, a linguist and business analyst.

Lee has been CEO of the ATM Industry Association (www.atmia.com), which has over 11,000 members in about 70 countries, since 2005. He is chairperson of the Consortium for Next Gen ATMs which has over 400 companies participating in this future-proofing exercise to link over 3 million ATMs with more than 5 billion mobile phones.

Michael is a qualified futurist, artist and writer living in Cape Town. In 2015, he published *Heartbeat*, a documentary novel about the world's first human heart transplant. His two works about understanding the social future through interdisciplinary causal analysis are *Knowing our Future* and *Codebreaking our Future*, both available on Amazon.com.

He has written two science fiction works, *Chrysalis*, a story about the world's first head transplant, and *Earthrise 2036*, a part-documentary, part-imaginary journey through the evolution of humanity from the rawest of origins in the Cradle of Humankind to the age of space exploration.

www.michaeljlee.com

TITLES BY THE AUTHOR

DOCUMENTARY NOVEL

Heartbeat

SCIENCE FICTION

Chrysalis

Earthrise 2036

POEMS

Three Hundred and Twenty-One Haiku

PLAYS

The Archive

NON-FICTION

Passage to Faith

A New Logic For Faith

The Courage to Believe

FUTURE STUDIES

Codebreaking our Future

Knowing our Future

www.beyondheads.com
www.michaeljlee.com
michael@positivedestiny.org

www.ingramcontent.com/pod-product-compliance
Lightning Source LLC
Chambersburg PA
CBHW032235050726
47591CB00001B/405